ZERO POINT WEIGHT LOSS COOKBOOK FOR BEGINNERS

Super Easy 0-Point Meals for Lasting Results
Without Guilt

Jacqueline Parish

Disclaimer

The information in this book is provided for educational purposes only. It is not intended as, nor should it be considered a substitute for, professional medical advice, diagnosis, or treatment. Always seek the advice of your physician or other qualified health provider with any questions you may have regarding a medical condition.

The Zero-Point Approach: What It Means and Why It Works

The zero-point approach to weight management represents a paradigm shift in how we think about food and dieting. This innovative method focuses on consuming foods that are nutrient-dense yet low in calories, allowing individuals to eat satisfying portions without strict calorie counting.

The core principle is straightforward: we assign zero points to certain foods, allowing us to consume them in reasonable quantities without tracking or measuring. Solid nutritional science forms the foundation of the zero-point approach. It leverages the concept of energy density, which refers to the number of calories in a given weight of food. Foods with low energy density provide fewer calories per gram, allowing for larger portions that promote satiety without excessive calorie intake.

This approach naturally steers individuals towards whole, unprocessed foods that are rich in fiber, protein, and water content—all factors that contribute to increased fullness and reduced overall calorie consumption.

Research has consistently shown that diets focusing on low-energy-dense foods lead to greater weight loss and improved long-term weight maintenance.

The American Journal of Clinical Nutrition published a study that revealed participants on a diet rich in low-energy-dense foods lost more weight and reported less hunger than those on a reduced-fat diet alone. This suggests that the zero-point approach not only aids in weight loss but also enhances dietary adherence by minimizing feelings of deprivation.

The effectiveness of the zero-point approach lies in its ability to reshape eating habits without imposing severe restrictions. By emphasizing nutrient-rich, whole foods, it naturally crowds out less healthy options and helps individuals develop a more balanced relationship with food. This stands in stark contrast to traditional, calorie-restricted diets, which often lead to cycles of deprivation and overeating.

Moreover, the zero-point approach aligns with the growing body of evidence supporting the importance of food quality over quantity. JAMA Internal Medicine published a landmark study demonstrating significant weight loss and improvements in metabolic health markers among individuals who focused on eating whole, unprocessed foods without calorie restrictions.

This underscores the power of choosing nutrient-dense foods, a cornerstone of the zero-point method.

One common misconception about the zero-point approach is that it promotes unlimited consumption of certain foods. In reality, it encourages mindful eating and portion awareness. Approach 6 emphasizes listening to hunger and fullness cues, allowing for the consumption of zero-point foods without strict measuring. This fosters a more intuitive relationship with eating, which research has shown to be beneficial for long-term weight management and overall health.

It's important to note that, while the zero-point approach is highly effective for many, individual responses may vary. Factors such as age, genetics, activity level, and overall health status can influence weight loss outcomes. However, the fundamental principles of this approach—emphasizing nutrient-dense, whole foods and promoting mindful eating—are universally beneficial for health and weight management.

Understanding Nutrient Density and Satiety

Nutrient density and satiety are two fundamental concepts that underpin the success of the zero-point approach to weight management. Understanding these principles is crucial for making informed food choices that support both health and weight loss goals.

Nutrient density is defined as the concentration of beneficial nutrients relative to a food's caloric content. Highly nutrient-dense foods provide substantial amounts of vitamins, minerals, fiber, and other essential nutrients with relatively few calories. These foods form the cornerstone of the zero-point approach, as they allow individuals to meet their nutritional needs while naturally limiting calorie intake. Examples of nutrient-dense foods include leafy greens, berries, cruciferous vegetables, lean proteins, and whole grains.

For instance, spinach offers high levels of vitamins A and K, folate, and iron with minimal calories. Similarly, salmon provides high-quality protein, omega-3 fatty acids, and vitamin D, contributing significantly to nutritional needs without excessive calorie loading.

The feeling of fullness and satisfaction after eating is called satiety. Foods that promote satiety play a crucial role in weight management by reducing overall calorie intake and minimizing between-meal snacking. The zero-point approach leverages this concept by emphasizing foods that are both nutrient-dense and satiating.

Factors Contributing to a Foods Satiating Power:
- **Protein:** High-protein foods increase satiety hormones and

reduce hunger stimulating hormones. Lean meats, fish, legumes, and eggs are excellent sources.

- **Fiber:** Foods rich in fiber slow digestion and promote fullness. Whole grains, vegetables, and fruits are fiber-rich options.

- **Water content:** Foods with high water content, such as soups and water-rich fruits, increase satiety by adding volume without calories.

- **Low energy density:** Foods that provide fewer calories per gram allow for larger, more satisfying portions.

The zero-point approach effectively combines nutrient density and satiety by promoting foods that excel in both aspects. For example, Greek yogurt is both nutrient-dense (providing protein, calcium, and probiotics) and satiating due to its protein content. Similarly, a mixed vegetable salad offers a variety of nutrients with fiber and water content that promotes fullness.

By focusing on these foods, individuals naturally reduce their calorie intake while meeting nutritional needs and feeling satisfied. This approach supports sustainable weight loss by creating a calorie deficit without the perception of deprivation often associated with traditional diets. Understanding and applying the concepts of nutrient density and satiety empowers individuals to make food choices that align with their health and weight management goals. It shifts the focus from restrictive eating to nourishing the body, fostering a positive and sustainable approach to nutrition and weight loss.

Stocking Your Pantry with Zero-Point Ingredients

A well-stocked pantry is the foundation of successful adherence to the zero-point approach. With a variety of nutritious, zero-point ingredients on hand, you'll be able to create satisfying meals with ease.

This guide will help you build a comprehensive pantry that supports your health goals while keeping both convenience and budget in mind.

Fruits and vegetables:

Fresh produce forms the cornerstone of the zero-point approach. Stock up on a variety of colorful fruits and vegetables to ensure a broad spectrum of nutrients.

- Berries (strawberries, blueberries, and raspberries): rich in antioxidants and fiber
- Citrus fruits (oranges, lemons, and limes): high in vitamin C and flavonoids
- Apples and pears: Provide pectin fiber for digestive health.
- Leafy greens (spinach, kale, and arugula): packed with vitamins and minerals
- Cruciferous vegetables (broccoli, cauliflower, Brussels sprouts): Offer cancer-fighting compounds.
- Bell peppers: excellent source of vitamin C and antioxidants
- Carrots and tomatoes: rich in beta-carotene and lycopene

Storage tip: Keep fruits and vegetables separate to prevent premature ripening. To control humidity levels, use produce drawers in your refrigerator.

Lean Proteins:

Protein is crucial for satiety and muscle maintenance. Include these lean options:

- Skinless chicken breast: Versatile and high in protein
- Turkey breast: Low in fat and rich in B vitamins
- Fish (cod, tilapia, salmon): Provides omega-3 fatty acids
- Egg whites: High-quality protein with minimal calories
- Non-fat Greek yogurt: Protein-rich and versatile for cooking

Storage tip: Keep raw meats on the bottom shelf of the refrigerator to prevent cross-contamination. Freeze portions for longer storage.

Legumes and Beans:
These plant-based proteins are fiber-rich and budget-friendly:
- Lentils: Quick-cooking and high in iron
- Chickpeas: Versatile for salads and homemade hummus
- Black beans: Rich in antioxidants and fiber
- Edamame: Complete protein source with all essential amino acids

Storage tip: Store dried legumes in airtight containers in a cool, dry place. Canned varieties offer convenience but rinse before use to reduce sodium content.

Herbs and Spices:
Enhance flavor without adding calories:
- Basil, oregano, thyme: Mediterranean flavors for vegetables and proteins
- Cumin, turmeric, coriander: Warming spices for curries and stews
- Cinnamon, nutmeg: Add sweetness without sugar to fruit dishes
- Garlic powder, onion powder: Convenient flavor boosters
- Red pepper flakes, black pepper: Add heat and metabolism-boosting properties

Storage tip: Store herbs and spices in airtight containers away from heat and light to preserve potency.

Pantry Staples:
These items provide the base for many zero-point meals:
- Vegetable broth: For soups and flavor-boosting
- Canned tomatoes: Versatile for sauces and stews

- Mustard Adds tang to dressings and marinades
- Vinegars (balsamic, apple cider): For dressings and flavor enhancement
- Unsweetened almond milk: Low-calorie base for smoothies

Storage tip: Check expiration dates regularly and practice the "first in, first out" method to minimize waste.

Meal Prep Strategies for Busy Beginners

Effective meal preparation is a cornerstone of success when following a zero-point diet, especially for busy individuals. By dedicating time to plan and prepare meals in advance, you can ensure that nutritious, zero-point options are always readily available.

This guide will provide you with practical strategies to streamline your meal prep process, save time, and support your health goals.

Time-Saving Techniques:
- **Batch Cooking:** Prepare larger quantities of staple ingredients like grilled chicken, roasted vegetables, or soup. These can be portioned and used throughout the week in various meals.
- **Use the "Cook Once, Eat Twice" Method:** When cooking dinner, make extra to use for lunch the next day. This doubles your efficiency with minimal extra effort.

- **Parallel Processing:** Multitask by having multiple items cooking simultaneously. For example, roast vegetables in the oven while grilling chicken and steaming rice on the stovetop.

- **Utilize Kitchen Appliances:** Slow cookers and Instant Pots can prepare meals with minimal hands-on time. Set them up in the morning for a ready-made dinner.

- **Pre-cut Vegetables:** Wash and chop vegetables for the week ahead. Store them in airtight containers for quick access during meal preparation.

- **Create a Salad Bar:** Prepare various salad ingredients and store them separately. This allows for quick assembly of fresh salads throughout the week.

Essential Kitchen Tools for Success

Basic Essentials:

- **Chef's Knife:** A high-quality chef's knife is indispensable for chopping vegetables, fruits, and lean proteins. It allows for precise cuts, improving both the texture and cooking time of your ingredients.

- **Cutting Boards:** Have at least two cutting boards – one for produce and another for proteins – to prevent cross-contamination. Opt for boards with juice grooves to contain liquids.

- **Measuring Cups and Spoons:** Essential for portion control and recipe accuracy. Look for durable, easy-to-clean sets with clear markings.

- **Digital Kitchen Scale:** Crucial for precise portion control, especially for proteins and higher-point ingredients. It helps maintain accuracy in your zero-point meal planning.

- **Non-Stick Skillet:** Perfect for cooking lean proteins and vegetables without added fats. Ensure it's oven-safe for versatility in cooking methods.

- **Large Pot:** Ideal for preparing soups, stews, and batch-cooking zero-point meals. A pot with a steamer insert adds versatility for steaming vegetables.

- **Blender:** Essential for making smoothies, pureed soups, and sauces. A high-powered blender can also handle tasks like grinding nuts for homemade nut butter.

- **Food Processor:** Useful for chopping vegetables, making cauliflower rice, and preparing homemade dips and sauces. It's a time-saver for meal prep.

- **Micro-plane Grater:** Perfect for zesting citrus fruits and grating ginger or garlic, adding flavor to dishes without extra calories.

- **Salad Spinner:** Ensures thoroughly washed and dried leafy greens, which is crucial for food safety and proper storage.

Optional Items for Enhanced Cooking:

- **Spiralizer:** Creates vegetable noodles, offering a low-calorie alternative to pasta in many dishes.

- **Air Fryer:** Provides a healthier method for achieving crispy textures without added oils.

- **Slow Cooker or Instant Pot:** Ideal for hands-off cooking of soups, stews, and lean proteins, saving time for busy individuals.

- **Immersion Blender:** Convenient for pureeing soups directly in the pot, reducing cleanup time.

- **Steamer Basket:** Allows for easy steaming of vegetables, preserving nutrients and flavor without added fats.

- **Silicone Baking Mats:** Provides a non-stick surface for roasting vegetables without oil, easy to clean and reusable.

- **Herb Scissors:** Efficiently chops fresh herbs, encouraging the use of these calorie-free flavor enhancers.

- **Citrus Juicer:** Extracts maximum juice from citrus fruits, useful for dressings and marinades.

These tools contribute to successful meal preparation by enhancing efficiency, ensuring proper portion control, and expanding the variety of cooking methods available.

Breakfast Recipes

Vanilla Berry Parfait with Chocolate Granola

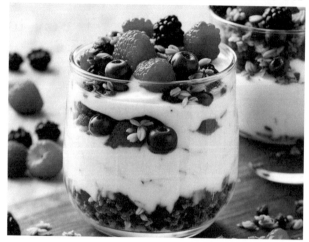

Serves: 1

Ingredients:

- 1 cup plain, unsweetened coconut yogurt
- ½ teaspoon vanilla extract Stevia or monk fruit, to taste
- 2 cups fresh or frozen berries of your choice
- ½ cup Chocolate Granola

Directions:

- In a medium bowl, combine yogurt, vanilla, and sweeten to taste. Top with berries and granola.

NUTRITION FACTS:

- CALORIES: 437

- PROTEINS: 9g
- CARBS: 67g
- FAT: 11g

Chocolate Granola

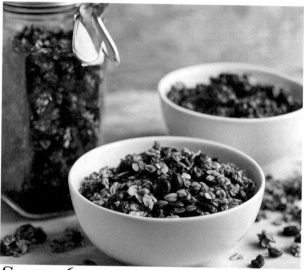

Serves: 6

Ingredients:

- 1½ cups (122g) rolled oats
- ¼ cup maple syrup
- 2 tablespoons unsweetened cocoa powder
- 1 teaspoon vanilla extract

Directions:

- Set the oven's temperature to 375°F. Lay parchment paper on a baking pan and set it aside.
- Put the oats, vanilla, cocoa powder, and maple syrup in a medium-sized bowl.

- Combine thoroughly. Once the baking sheet has been prepared, distribute the mixture evenly and bake for 10 minutes, or until it is lightly browned.
- Let the granola cool fully before putting it in an airtight jar to keep it fresh for up to a week at room temperature.

NUTRITION FACTS:
- CALORIES: 117
- PROTEIN: 3g
- CARBS: 21g
- FAT: 2g

Raspberry Chocolate Muffins

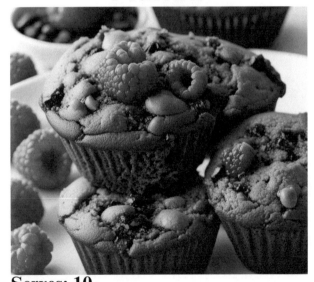

Serves: 10

Ingredients:
- Cooking spray
- 1 cup water
- 1 teaspoon vanilla extract
- 1½ cups (180g) whole-wheat flour, or oat flour for gluten-free muffins
- ¼ cup (50g) sugar
- 1 teaspoon baking powder
- ¼ teaspoon sea salt
- 1 cup fresh raspberries
- ¼ cup dairy-free chocolate chips

Directions:
- Set the oven's temperature to 375°F. Grease nine or ten silicone muffin pan cups lightly with cooking spray, then set them aside.
- Mix the water and vanilla together in a big mixing bowl.
- Add the flour, sugar, baking powder, salt and mix together until a homogeneous mixture is achieved.
- Add the chocolate chips and raspberries and fold gently until they are uniformly distributed.
- Evenly distribute the batter, about ¼ cup each muffin cup, among the prepared muffin cups.
- A toothpick put into the center of a muffin should come out clean after 15 to 18 minutes of baking (apart from any melted

chocolate or raspberry).

- Let the muffins cool fully before storing them for up to three days at room temperature in an airtight container.

NUTRITION FACTS:

- CALORIES: 362
- PROTEIN: 9g
- CARBS: 60g
- FAT: 7.5g

Blueberry Lemon Oat Waffles

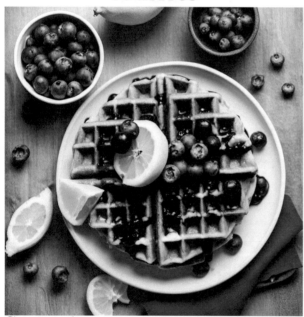

Serves: 1

Ingredients:

- Cooking spray
- 1 cup (82g) rolled oats
- 1 medium ripe banana (101g)
- 1 teaspoon vanilla extract
- ½ teaspoon lemon extract
- ½ teaspoon baking powder
- Pinch of sea salt
- ¾ cup water
- ½ cup whole fresh blueberries, plus ½ cup mashed and warmed blueberries, for serving
- 1 tablespoon maple syrup, for serving

Directions:

- For this dish, I use a four-waffle iron, so preheat it and give it a quick spritz of cooking spray.
- Put the oats, banana, baking powder, vanilla, lemon extract, and salt in a blender. Puree until smooth after adding the water.
- Add the ½ cup of whole blueberries and fold gently.
- Using about ¼ cup of batter for each waffle, pour the batter into the waffle iron.
- This should be done in two batches if you're using a four-waffle iron.
- Cook the waffles for 5 to 8 minutes, or until they stop sticking and separating.
- Continue with the leftover batter, then serve hot with the mashed blueberries and syrup.

NUTRITION FACTS:

- CALORIES: 459
- PROTEIN: 12g
- CARBS: 77g
- FAT: 6g

Strawberry Lemon Muffins

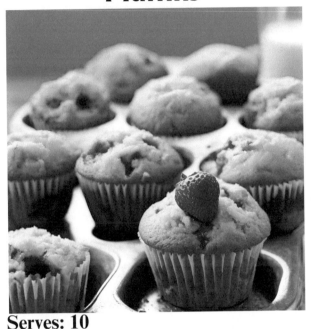

Serves: 10

Ingredients:

- Cooking spray
- 1½ cups (180g) whole-wheat flour, or oat flour for gluten-free muffins
- ¼ cup (50g) sugar
- 1 teaspoon baking powder
- ¼ teaspoon sea salt
- 1 cup water
- 1 teaspoon vanilla extract
- 1 teaspoon lemon extract
- 1 cup hulled and chopped fresh strawberries
- 1 teaspoon lemon zest

Directions:

- Set the oven's temperature to 375°F. Grease ten muffin tin wells with cooking spray, then set them aside.
- Combine the flour, sugar, baking powder, and salt in a medium-sized bowl using a whisk. Put aside.
- Combine the water, vanilla, and lemon extract in a small bowl.
- The water mixture should be added to the dry ingredients gradually and mixed until smooth. Stir in the lemon zest and strawberries gently.
- Spoon about ¼ cup of batter into each of the muffin cups that have been prepped.
- Bake for 18 to 22 minutes, or until a toothpick inserted into the center of a muffin comes out clean.
- Let the muffins cool fully before taking them out of the pan.
- The muffins can be stored for up to three days at room temperature in an airtight container.

Strawberry Lemon Muffins

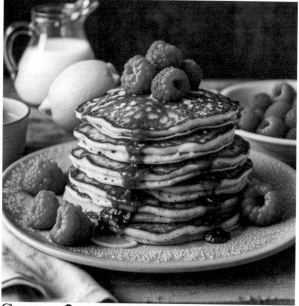

Serves: 2

Ingredients:
- 1¼ cups (150g) whole-wheat flour, or oat flour for gluten-free pancakes
- 2 tablespoons (25g) sugar
- 2 teaspoons baking powder
- ½ teaspoon sea salt
- 1¼ cups water
- 1 teaspoon vanilla extract
- 1 teaspoon lemon extract
- 1 teaspoon lemon zest
- ½ tablespoon poppy seeds
- 1 cup fresh raspberries, halved, plus more for serving (optional)
- Cooking spray (optional)
- Maple syrup, for serving

Directions:
- Combine the flour, sugar, baking powder, and salt in a medium-sized bowl. Put aside.
- Combine the water, vanilla, and lemon extract in a small bowl.
- Add the water mixture to the dry ingredients gradually while stirring, and whisk until smooth.
- Add the raspberries, poppy seeds, and zest of the lemon and fold gently.
- Turn up the heat to medium-high in a big nonstick skillet.
- You can use cooking spray to ensure consistent cooking, but it's optional.
- Divide the batter into the pan using a ¼-cup scoop while working in batches.
- Cook for two to three minutes, or until the bottom of the pancake is light gold. Repeat on the opposite side after flipping.

- Proceed with the remaining batter and proceed to serve the pancakes hot, garnishing them with syrup and raspberries if preferred.

NUTRITION FACTS:
- CALORIES: 360
- PROTEIN: 11g
- CARBS: 63g
- FAT: 3g

Blueberry Peach Crisp

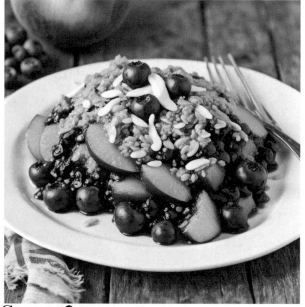

Serves: 2

Ingredients:

For The Filling:
- 4 cups (300g) fresh or frozen and thawed blueberries
- 4 peaches (350g), sliced, or 4 cups thawed frozen peach slices
- 4 tablespoons fresh lemon juice
- 4 teaspoons vanilla extract

For The Toppings:
- 1 cup (41g) rolled oats
- 2 tablespoons maple syrup
- 1 teaspoon vanilla extract
- ½ teaspoon almond extract

Directions:
- Set the oven's temperature to 375°F.
- Prepare the filling: Combine the peaches, blueberries, lemon juice, and vanilla in a medium-sized bowl.
- Split the mixture between two dishes measuring 6 by 8 inches. Put aside.
- Prepare the topping by combining the oats, almond extract, vanilla, and maple syrup in a medium-sized bowl.
- Evenly divide the mixture, then pour it over the two-fruit bowls.
- Bake for 20 minutes, or until the fruit bubbles and the topping is golden brown.

NUTRITION FACTS:
- CALORIES: 543
- PROTEIN: 11g
- CARBS: 102g
- FAT: 2g

Breakfast Salad

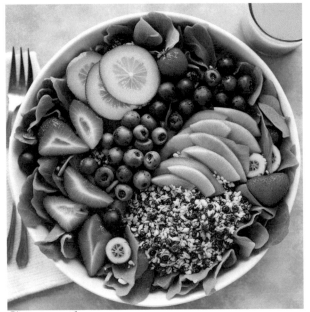

Serves: 1

Ingredients:

For The Citrus Poppy Seed Dressing:

- ¼ cup fresh orange juice
- 1 tablespoon fresh lime juice
- 1 teaspoon maple syrup or other sweetener of your choice
- ¼ teaspoon poppy seeds

For The Salad:

- 4 cups spring greens or other greens you like
- 1 peach, pit removed and sliced
- 1 cup hulled and chopped strawberries
- ¾ cup blueberries
- 1 cup (260g) cooked or canned white beans or chickpeas (drained and rinsed if canned); optional
- 1 tablespoon chopped fresh mint leaves (optional)

Directions:

- To make the dressing, combine the orange juice, lime juice, poppy seeds, maple syrup, or other preferred sweetener in a small bowl. Put aside.
- Prepare the salad: Arrange the greens in a big bowl, then add the peach slices, blueberries, and strawberries on top.
- Garnish with beans or chickpeas and mint, if desired.
- Add the dressing to the salad and toss to coat (I use the entire amount).

NUTRITION FACTS:

- CALORIES: 456
- PROTEIN: 21g
- CARBS: 68g
- FAT: 1.7g

Lemon Berry Patch Yogurt

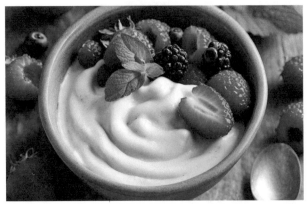

Serves: 1

Ingredients:

- 1 ½ cups plain, unsweetened coconut yogurt
- ½ teaspoon lemon extract, plus more to taste
- Stevia or monk fruit sweetener, to taste
- 1½ cups sliced strawberries
- ¾ cup fresh or frozen and defrosted raspberries
- ¾ cup fresh or frozen and defrosted blueberries
- ¾ cup fresh or frozen and defrosted blackberries

Directions:

- Whisk together the yogurt and lemon extract in a medium-sized bowl.
- If preferred, enhance the taste by adding additional lemon extract and sweeten to personal preference.
- Place the berries on top, then savor.

NUTRITION FACTS:

- CALORIES: 389
- PROTEIN: 6g
- CARBS: 48g
- FAT: 13g

Chocolate Peanut Butter Oatmeal

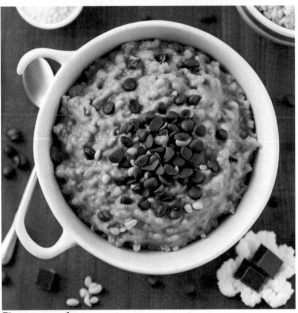

Serves: 1

Ingredients:

- 1½ cups plus 1 tablespoon water
- ¾ cup rolled oats
- ½ cup frozen riced cauliflower
- ¼ teaspoon vanilla extract, plus more to taste
- Stevia or monk fruit, to taste
- 2 tablespoons powdered peanut butter
- 2 tablespoons dairy-free chocolate chips

Directions:

- Place the riced cauliflower, oats, and 1½ cups of water in a medium pot.
- Over medium-high heat, bring

the mixture to a boil while stirring from time to time.

- Then, lower the heat right away to a simmer. Stir and simmer for a further 3 to 5 minutes, or until the oats are soft.
- Add the vanilla and, if desired, add additional vanilla. Sweeten to taste with stevia or monk fruit.
- Combine the powdered peanut butter with the remaining 1 tablespoon of water in a small bowl and whisk until smooth.
- Sprinkle the chocolate chips and peanut butter over the oats and serve.

NUTRITION FACTS:

- CALORIES: 455
- PROTEIN: 17g
- CARBS: 56g
- FAT: 15g

Pineapple Ginger Smoothie

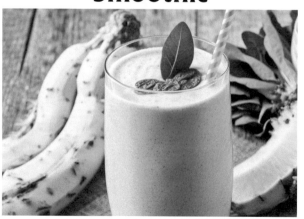

Serves: 1
Ingredients:

- 2 medium bananas (236g)
- 1½ cups (280g) frozen pineapple
- 2 handfuls of spinach
- ½-inch piece of ginger, peeled
- 1 cup plain, unsweetened almond milk

Directions:

- Put the bananas, pineapple, spinach, ginger, and almond milk in a blender. Process till smooth.

NUTRITION FACTS:

- CALORIES: 436
- PROTEIN: 8g
- CARBS: 86g
- FAT: 3.5g

Chocolate Peanut Butter Smoothie

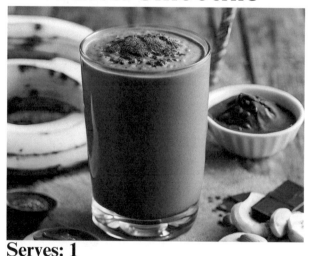

Serves: 1
Ingredients:

- 2 medium bananas (236g)
- 1 cup plain, unsweetened almond milk
- ½ cup (41g) rolled oats
- 2 tablespoons (12g) powdered peanut butter
- 1 tablespoon unsweetened cocoa powder
- ½ teaspoon vanilla extract

Directions:
- In a blender, blend together the bananas, almond milk, oats, powdered peanut butter, chocolate powder, vanilla, and half to one cup of ice cubes.
- Process till smooth.

NUTRITION FACTS:
- CALORIES: 468
- PROTEIN: 15g
- CARBS: 78g
- FAT: 8g

Coffee Caramel Smoothie

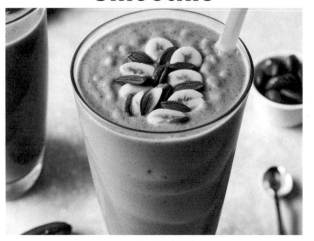

Serves: 1

Ingredients:
- 3 medium frozen bananas (354g), roughly chopped
- 1½ cups plain, unsweetened almond milk
- 2 Medjool dates, pitted, plus
- ½ Medjool date, pitted and chopped, for serving (optional) (48g)
- 2 teaspoons instant coffee (decaf, if preferred), plus more to taste (if you want stronger coffee flavor)
- ½ teaspoon vanilla extract
- 1 teaspoon dairy-free chocolate chips, for serving (optional)

Directions:
- Put the bananas, almond milk, Medjool dates, instant coffee, and vanilla in a high-speed blender. Process till smooth.
- If preferred, sprinkle chocolate chips and the chopped date on top.

NUTRITION FACTS:
- CALORIES: 502
- PROTEIN: 6g
- CARBS: 108g
- FAT: 5g

Fruit Salsa with Cinnamon Toast

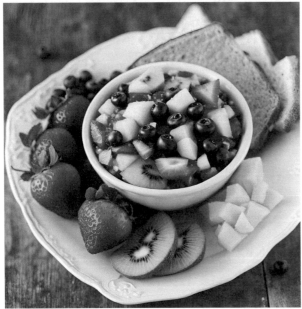

Serves: 1

Ingredients:

For The Fruit Salsa:

- 1 cup chopped strawberries
- 1 cup diced mango
- ½ cup blueberries
- ½ cup diced kiwi

For The Cinnmon Toast:

- 2 slices of sprouted whole-grain bread
- 1 teaspoon sugar
- ¼ teaspoon ground cinnamon

Directions:

- Prepare the fruit salsa by combining all of the fruit in a medium-sized bowl and tossing gently to thoroughly combine. Put aside.

- Prepare the cinnamon toast: Toast the bread in a toaster or toaster oven until it reaches your desired level of doneness.
- In a separate small bowl, combine sugar and cinnamon.
- Once the bread is cooked, evenly distribute the cinnamon-sugar mixture over both pieces.
- Cut the toast into squares and top with the fruit salsa.

NUTRITION FACTS:

- CALORIES: 438
- PROTEIN: 12g
- CARBS: 82g
- FAT: 3g

Mushroom Steak and Eggs with Herby Caesar

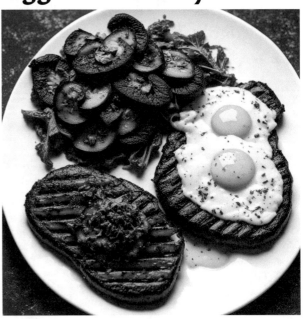

Serves: 1

Ingredients:

FOR THE STEAKS

- ¼ cup vegan Worcestershire sauce
- ¼ cup water
- 1 teaspoon minced garlic
- ¼ teaspoon liquid smoke
- ⅛ teaspoon onion powder
- Freshly ground black pepper, to taste
- 2 large portobello mushroom caps (8 ounces), wiped clean.
- Cooking spray (optional)

FOR SERVING

- 3 Garden Vegetable Chickpea Omelets, warmed
- 5 tablespoons Lemon-Herb Caesar
- Minced fresh chives, for garnish

Directions:

- To prepare the steaks, whisk together the Worcestershire sauce, water, onion powder, garlic, liquid smoke, and a few grinds of black pepper in a shallow bowl.
- Add the mushrooms and stir to ensure that they are evenly coated with the marinade. Give the mushrooms ten minutes to marinate at room temperature.
- Turn up the heat to medium-high in a large nonstick skillet.

- You can use cooking spray if you'd like to help the mushrooms brown, but it's not necessary.
- Cook the mushrooms, top side down, for 3 to 5 minutes or until they brown. You can add a little water if they start to stick.
- Repeat on the opposite side after flipping. Put aside.

Assemble:

- Cut the omelettes into pieces that resemble scrambled eggs.
- Next, slice the mushrooms and place them on top of the eggs.
- Drizzle the vinaigrette over the mushrooms and garnish with chives.

NUTRITION FACTS:

- CALORIES: 367
- PROTEIN: 16g
- CARBS: 41g
- FAT: 12g

Garden Vegetable Chickpea Omelet

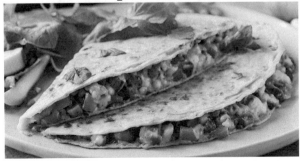

Serves: 1

Ingredients:

- 1 cup (92g) chickpea flour
- 1 cup water
- ¼ teaspoon garlic powder
- ⅛ teaspoon onion powder
- ½ teaspoon black salt or sea salt
- Pinch of turmeric (optional, for color)
- Cooking spray (optional)
- Assorted veggies
- Garlic salt, to taste
- ¼ medium avocado (25g)
- Your favorite salsa and/or hot sauce, for serving

Directions:

- Combine the chickpea flour, water, onion and garlic powders, sea or black salt, and turmeric (if using) in a medium-sized bowl.
- The batter for the omelette needs to be smooth. Put aside.
- Turn up the heat to medium-high in a large nonstick skillet.
- You can use cooking spray to ensure consistent cooking, but it's optional.
- Cook the vegetables with a touch of garlic salt until soft.
- The timing varies based on the quantity and type of vegetables.
- If vegetables become stuck, add a splash of water to the pan to release them.
- Transfer the vegetables to a plate or bowl, then clean the pan.
- If preferred, reapply cooking spray to the pan and set it over medium heat.
- Using a measuring cup measuring ½ cup, scoop the batter into the pan.
- Gently spread the batter using the bottom of the measuring cup until it takes the shape of a big pancake, about 6 inches in diameter and ¼ inch thick.
- Cook for about 3 minutes, or until the bottom begins to brown and the centre is no longer wet.
- Cook for a further three minutes after flipping, or until the other side is firm and faintly browned.
- Spoon the omelette onto a plate, then repeat with the rest of the batter.
- Spoon the vegetables into each omelette and garnish with salsa, avocado, and/or spicy sauce.

- Serve right away.

NUTRITION FACTS:
- CALORIES: 359
- PROTEIN: 21g
- CARBS: 44g
- FAT: 6g

Garlic Herb Potato Waffles

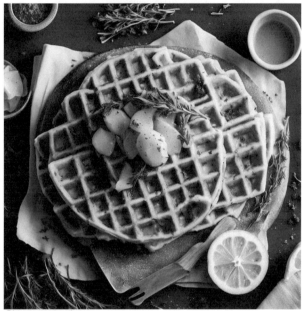

Serves: 1

Ingredients:
- 2 medium to large Yukon Gold potatoes (550g)
- 2 teaspoons dried rosemary
- 1 teaspoon garlic powder
- ½ teaspoon onion powder
- ½ teaspoon dried thyme
- ½ teaspoon sea salt Cooking spray
- 3 tablespoons Lemon-Herb Caesar, Smokehouse Ranch, or
- Pimento Cheese Sauce, optional

Directions:
- Steam or bake potatoes without peeling them.
- Preheat the oven to 425°F if you plan to bake.
- Pierce the potatoes on all sides and bake them on a baking sheet for 45 minutes, or until they are fork tender.
- Cut the potatoes into 1-inch cubes and place them in a medium-sized or big pot if you plan to boil them.
- Place the potatoes in a pot with just enough water to cover them, cover the saucepan, and bring the mixture to a boil over medium-high heat.
- Boil until fork-tender, 20 to 25 minutes.
- If utilising an Instant Pot, place the potatoes inside the steaming basket. Place the lid on after adding just enough water to cover.
- For eighteen minutes, cook using the Steam option.
- Manually release the pressure.
- Let the potatoes cool before heating up a waffle iron to a

high temperature.

- Once potatoes have cooled, combine with rosemary, garlic powder, onion powder, thyme, and salt in a larger bowl.
- Mash the potatoes with a fork or potato masher until they are fairly smooth (a few lumps are acceptable), then mix in the seasonings thoroughly.
- Apply a thin layer of cooking spray to the waffle iron.
- Use one-third of the potato mixture to make patties, which you then put in the waffle iron.
- Cook until crispy, 5 to 10 minutes.
- After the waffle is done, transfer it to a plate and continue with the leftover potato mixture.
- You should have three waffles in the end.
- Savour warm, topped with your preferred sauce.

NUTRITION FACTS:
- CALORIES: 433
- PROTEIN: 10g
- CARBS: 88g
- FAT: 1g

Gardener's Breakfast

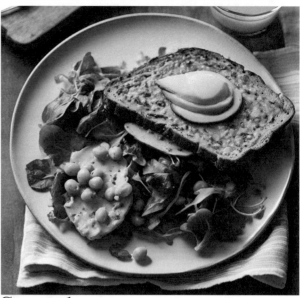

Serves: 1

Ingredients:
- ½ tablespoon maple syrup
- ½ tablespoon fresh lemon juice
- ½ tablespoon Dijon mustard
- 3 cups spring greens
- 2 Garden Vegetable Chickpea Omelets, warmed
- 1 slice sprouted grain bread, toasted
- ¼ avocado (25g), smashed
- ¼ teaspoon everything bagel seasoning
- Pinch of sprouts of your choice

Directions:
- Combine the Dijon, lemon juice, and maple syrup in a small bowl. Mix well and whisk until smooth.
- Put the greens in a big platter

and pour the dressing over them.

- Toss together, then place the omelettes on top of the greens.
- Spread avocado on the toast and sprinkle with everything bagel seasoning. Place the sprouts on top and serve with the omelettes and greens.

NUTRITION FACTS:

- CALORIES: 297
- PROTEIN: 15g
- CARBS: 37g
- FAT: 7

Egg and Avocado Breakfast Sandwich

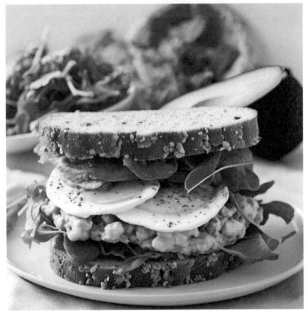

Serves: 1

Ingredients:

- 1 tablespoon coarse-ground Dijon mustard
- 2 slices of sprouted whole-grain bread
- 2 tablespoons hummus
- 1 Garden Vegetable Chickpea Omelets
- 1 cup greens of your choice (I love arugula for this)
- ½ small avocado (50g), sliced
- Sprouts (optional)
- Hot sauce, salsa, or ¼ cup Tzatziki Sauce (or store-bought)

Directions:

- Combine the Dijon, lemon juice, and maple syrup in a small bowl. Mix well and whisk until smooth.
- Put the greens in a big platter
- Top one slice of bread with hummus and top the other with mustard.
- Arrange the omelette, greens, avocado, and sprouts (if used) on top of the hummus.
- Add a drizzle of spicy sauce, salsa, or tzatziki, then place the second slice of bread on top.

NUTRITION FACTS:

- CALORIES: 377
- PROTEIN: 16g
- CARBS: 39g
- FAT: 10g

Breakfast Tacos

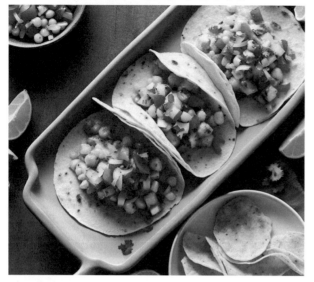

Serves: 1

Ingredients:

- Cooking spray
- 1 small Yukon Gold potato (154g), shredded
- ½ cup diced red bell pepper
- ¼ cup diced yellow onion
- Garlic salt, to taste
- 1 Garden Vegetable Chickpea Omelet, chopped
- 3 (6-inch) corn tortillas
- ½ cup Pico de Gallo, or salsa of your choice
- ¼ small avocado (25g), peeled, pitted, and thinly sliced

Directions:

- Turn up the heat to medium-high in a medium nonstick skillet.
- Coat the pan lightly with cooking spray before adding the potato, pepper, and onion.
- Add a dash of garlic salt for seasoning, and cook for three to five minutes, or until the potatoes are tender and the vegetables are starting to brown.
- Stir in the chopped Garden Vegetable Chickpea Omelette to the pan and simmer until it is fully heated, which should take approximately one minute.
- Spoon the veggie and omelette mixture over each tortilla, garnish with avocado and Pico de Gallo, and savour.

NUTRITION FACTS:

- CALORIES: 435
- PROTEIN: 13g
- CARBS: 70g
- FAT: 7.5g

Lunch and Dinner Recipes

Sweet Potato Black Bean Curry

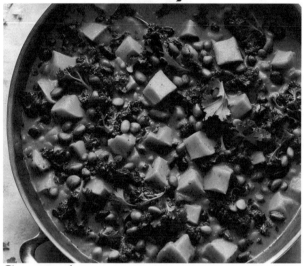

Serves: 1

Ingredients:

- 1 medium sweet potato (250g)
- ¼ cup diced yellow onion
- 1 cup unsweetened almond milk
- ¾ cup canned light coconut milk
- 3 teaspoons yellow curry paste, plus more to taste
- 2 cups chopped kale leaves
- ¼ cup canned black beans, drained and rinsed
- 1 teaspoon fresh lime juice
- ½ teaspoon sea salt, plus more to taste
- Stevia or maple syrup, to taste
- ½ cup packed fresh cilantro, chopped
- 1 cup steamed white rice, for serving

Directions:

- Set the oven's temperature to 425°F. Put parchment paper on a baking pan.
- Pierce the sweet potato all over with a fork.
- Place the potato on the baking sheet that has been preheated and bake for 40 minutes, or until a knife can easily slides in.
- When the potato has cooled a little, peel and discard the skin with your hands.
- Chop the potato into small chunks. Put aside.
- Sauté the onions in a medium pot over medium-high heat for about 3 minutes, or until they start to brown.
- Stir in the almond milk, coconut milk, and curry paste until thoroughly combined.
- Add the kale, beans, lime juice, and salt.

- Cook, stirring, for about 5 minutes, or until the kale has wilted and everything is thoroughly cooked.
- If necessary, add a few drops of stevia and/or more salt to season.
- Serve over rice after adding the cilantro.

NUTRITION FACTS:
- CALORIES: 623 y
- PROTEIN: 15g
- CARBS: 93g
- FAT: 14g

Lemon Chickpea Soup

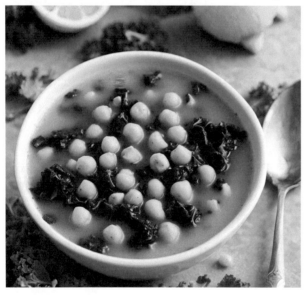

Serves: 1
Ingredients:
- 1 (15-ounce) can chickpeas, drained and rinsed
- ½ small yellow onion (110g), diced
- 2 vegan bouillon cubes, plus more to taste
- 1 tablespoon minced garlic
- Juice of 1 lemon
- 1 teaspoon dried oregano
- 4 cups water
- 1½ cups chopped kale leaves
- 1 cup plain, unsweetened plant-based milk
- Garlic salt, to taste
- Freshly ground black pepper, to taste
- Chopped fresh parsley, for garnish

Directions:
- The chickpeas, onion, garlic, bouillon cubes, lemon juice, and oregano should all be combined in a medium-sized pot over medium heat.
- After adding the water, stir and cook the mixture.
- Cook for 10 minutes until the soup is thoroughly cooked and the flavours have combined.
- After turning off the heat, add the kale and give it two minutes to wilt.
- Add the milk, stir, and season with pepper and garlic salt to taste.
- Add parsley as a garnish and

proceed to serve.

NUTRITION FACTS:

- CALORIES: 474
- PROTEIN: 21g
- CARBS: 46g
- FAT: 16g

Potato Kale Soup

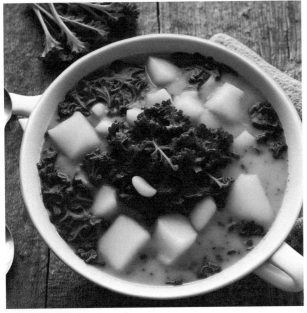

Serves: 2

Ingredients:

- Cooking spray
- 1 medium yellow onion
- 1 tablespoon minced garlic
- 1 large Yukon gold potato (400g), diced
- 1 (15-ounce) can (245g) white beans, drained and rinsed
- 2 vegan bouillon cubes
- 6 cups water
- 1 bunch of kale leaves (120g), chopped (6 cups)
- 1 cup plain, unsweetened almond milk
- 1 teaspoon chili flakes
- 1½ teaspoon garlic salt, or more to taste

Directions:

- Turn up the heat to medium in a medium saucepan.
- You can use cooking spray to ensure consistent cooking, but it's optional.
- Add the onion and simmer for 3 to 4 minutes, or until softened.
- You can add a little water if it begins to stick.
- Add the garlic and sauté for one minute, or until it is fragrant and not yet beginning to brown.
- Stir in the water after adding the potato, white beans, and bouillon cubes.
- Cook for 15 minutes, uncovered, until potatoes are fork tender.
- Remove from heat and add kale and almond milk. Stir well.
- After a few minutes of wilting, add the chilli flakes and season with garlic salt to taste.

NUTRITION FACTS:

- CALORIES: 436g
- PROTEIN: 20g
- CARBS: 62g
- FAT: 6g

Lentil Mushroom Stew

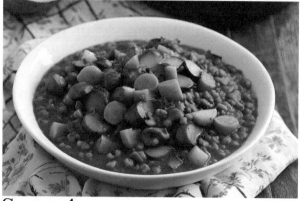

Serves: 4

Ingredients:

- Cooking spray
- 16 ounces baby bella mushrooms, wiped clean and quartered
- 1 medium yellow onion, chopped
- 1 cup peeled and diced carrots (3 medium carrots)
- 3 garlic cloves, minced
- 2 medium russet or Yukon Gold potatoes (426g), cut into 1- inch pieces
- 1 (14-ounce) can or jar tomato sauce
- 1 cup dry brown lentils (208g)
- 3 vegan bouillon cubes
- 1 dried bay leaf,

- 1 teaspoon sea salt
- ½ teaspoon dried oregano
- Freshly ground black pepper, to taste
- 3 cups water
- 1 cup plain, unsweetened almond milk
- Fresh parsley, chopped, to garnish

Directions:

- If utilising an Instant Pot, place the mushrooms, onion, carrots, and garlic in the pot and turn it to the Sauté option.
- Cook for 5 to 8 minutes, stirring frequently, or until the vegetables are soft.
- Include the lentils, potatoes, tomato sauce, bay leaf, bouillon cubes, salt, oregano, and a few grinds of pepper. Add the water and stir.
- Put the cover on tight, cook for 15 minutes under high pressure, and then let the pressure drop naturally. (This usually takes a total of forty minutes.)
- Take off the cover, throw away the bay leaf, and mix in the almond milk.
- Taste and adjust the seasonings accordingly, then add the

parsley as a garnish.

- For stovetop preparation, preheat a medium-sized or large pot over medium-high heat.
- You can use cooking spray to ensure consistent cooking, but it's optional.
- Add the garlic, onion, carrots, and mushrooms. Sauté for 5 to 8 minutes, stirring frequently, or until the veggies are tender.
- A quick spray of water can be added if the veggies begin to stick.
- Include the potatoes, lentils, tomato sauce, bay leaf, bouillon cubes, salt, oregano, and a few grinds of pepper.
- After adding the water, stir and cook the mixture.
- Sauté the potatoes for 15 to 20 minutes, or until they are soft, while covered and tossing from time to time.
- Take out and throw away the bay leaf before adding the almond milk.
- Taste and adjust the seasonings.
- Garnish with the chopped parsley and serve.

NUTRITION FACTS:

- CALORIES: 384
- PROTEIN: 22g
- CARBS: 55g
- FAT: 4g

Potato Corn Chowder

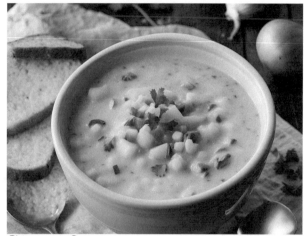

Serves: 2

Ingredients:

- 1 medium yellow onion, chopped
- ½ cup chopped celery (about 2 medium stalks)
- 3 garlic cloves, minced
- 2 medium to large russet potatoes (455g), peeled and diced
- 3 vegan bouillon cubes
- 3 cups water
- 1 cup plain, unsweetened almond milk
- ¼ cup cornstarch
- 1 (15-ounce) can corn kernels, drained, or 1 ¼ cups fresh or frozen corn kernels

- ¼ cup chopped fresh parsley leaves, for serving
- Sea salt and freshly ground black pepper, to taste

Directions:

- Combine the onion and celery in a medium or large pot.
- For three to four minutes, or until the onions start to soften, sauté over medium-high heat.
- Add the garlic and simmer for about a minute, or until it is aromatic and starting to soften.
- Include the potatoes, water, and bouillon cubes; heat to a boil.
- Lower the heat to a simmer and cook, uncovered, stirring now and then, for about 15 minutes, or until the potatoes are fork-tender.
- In the meantime, mix the starch and almond milk into a slurry in a small bowl. Once potatoes are soft, add almond milk slurry and corn to the soup.
- Raise the temperature to medium-high, cook for one minute.
- The consistency of the soup should be similar to gravy.
- Take the saucepan off of the burner, add the parsley and adjust the seasoning with salt and pepper.
- Serve warm.

NUTRITION FACTS:

- CALORIES: 405
- PROTEIN: 10g
- CARBS: 75g
- FAT: 7g

Falafel Cauliflower Pitas

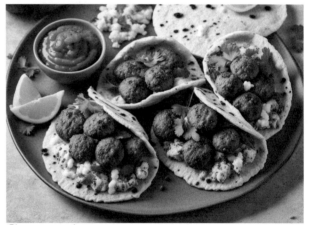

Serves: 1

Ingredients:

- 4 cups cauliflower florets, cut into bite-size pieces
- Juice of ½ lemon
- 1 teaspoon ground coriander
- ¾ teaspoon garlic salt
- ½ teaspoon ground cumin
- ¼ teaspoon chili powder (optional)
- ¼ teaspoon ground turmeric
- ¼ teaspoon freshly ground black pepper
- Pinch of ground cinnamon

- Cooking spray
- 3 low-calorie pitas
- 1 cup spring greens or chopped romaine, Bibb, or butter lettuce
- 1 medium Roma tomato, sliced
- ½ small cucumber, sliced
- ¼ cup sliced red onion
- ½ cup Tzatziki Sauce
- 1 tablespoon chopped fresh parsley leaves
- 1 tablespoon chopped fresh cilantro leaves

Directions:

- Set the oven's temperature to 425°F. Place parchment paper on a baking pan and set it aside.
- Put the cauliflower, lemon juice, coriander, garlic salt, cumin, turmeric, pepper, cinnamon, chili powder (if using), and coriander in a big bowl. Toss to thoroughly coat the cauliflower.
- Pour the batter onto the baking sheet that has been ready and level it out into a single layer.
- Apply a thin layer of cooking spray to the cauliflower to aid in its crisping while roasting.
- Roast the cauliflower for 20 to 25 minutes, or until it starts to turn brown.
- Take out of the oven and let the cauliflower cool a little.
- Distribute the cauliflower among the three pitas and top with the onion, tomato, cucumber, and greens.
- Sprinkle the parsley and cilantro on top of each pita and cover with ¼ cup of Tzatziki Sauce.

NUTRITION FACTS:

- CALORIES: 405
- PROTEIN: 29g
- CARBS: 44g
- FAT: 9g

Samosa Wraps

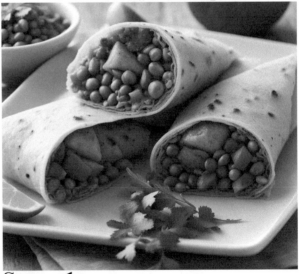

Serves: 1

Ingredients:

- 1 large Yukon Gold potato (330g)
- ¼ cup fresh or frozen peas

- 1 tablespoon chopped fresh cilantro leaves
- 1 teaspoon fresh lime juice
- ½ teaspoon curry powder
- ½ teaspoon garlic powder
- ¼ teaspoon onion powder
- ¼ teaspoon sea salt
- 2 low-calorie wraps
- 1 medium Roma tomato, sliced
- 4 cups greens

Directions:

- Set the oven's temperature to 425°F. After piercing the potato all over, bake it for 45 minutes on a baking sheet, or until it is fork-tender.
- Let the potato cool slightly while you prepare the peas.
- A few inches of water should be simmered over medium heat in a small or medium pot. After adding the peas, cook for 30 seconds or until they are soft and bright green. Transfer peas to a bowl and set aside.
- Move the potato to a medium-sized bowl and mash it smooth with a fork or potato masher.
- Mix thoroughly to incorporate the peas, cilantro, lime juice, curry powder, garlic powder, onion powder, and salt.

- Fill each of the two wraps with half of the potato mixture.
- Place the tomato and greens on top, fold the wraps, and enjoy!

NUTRITION FACTS:

- CALORIES: 489
- PROTEIN: 28g
- CARBS: 75g
- FAT: 5g

Herby White Bean Sammy

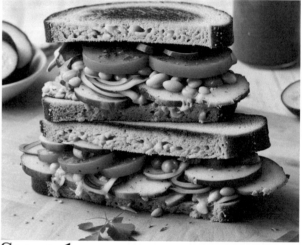

Serves: 1

Ingredients:

- 2 slices sprouted whole-grain bread, toasted
- ½ cup Herby Bean Dip
- 2 tablespoons Smokehouse Ranch
- 1 medium carrot, shredded
- 1 small tomato, sliced
- ½ small cucumber, sliced
- ¼ medium avocado (25g),

- 1 tablespoon chopped fresh cilantro leaves
- 1 teaspoon fresh lime juice
- ½ teaspoon curry powder
- ½ teaspoon garlic powder
- ¼ teaspoon onion powder
- ¼ teaspoon sea salt
- 2 low-calorie wraps
- 1 medium Roma tomato, sliced
- 4 cups greens peeled, pitted, and sliced
- ¼ cup sliced red onion
- ¼ cup sprouts of your choice
- 2 lettuce leaves of your choice

Directions:

- Drizzle the Smokehouse Ranch over a toasted slice of bread after spreading the Herby Bean Dip over it.
- Add the avocado, tomato, cucumber, carrot, onion, sprouts, lettuce leaves, and second slice of bread on top.

NUTRITION FACTS:

- CALORIES: 465
- PROTEIN: 23g
- CARBS: 56g
- FAT: 10g

Apple Pimento Grilled Cheese with Caramelized Onions and Arugula

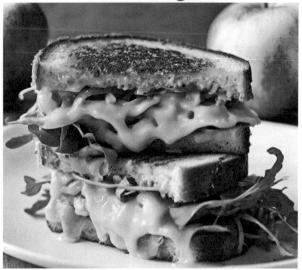

Serves: 2

Ingredients:

- 1 small sweet yellow onion, sliced
- ⅛ teaspoon garlic salt
- 4 slices sprouted whole-grain bread
- ½ cup Pimento Cheese Sauce
- 1 small Honeycrisp apple, cored and sliced
- 1 cup arugula

Directions:

- To a medium-sized or large nonstick pan, add the onions and season with the garlic salt.
- Allow the onions to brown for two to three minutes on one

- side without stirring over medium-high heat.
- Stir them and continue to brown for a further two to three minutes, or until they are tender and golden.
- Wipe clean the pan after transferring the onions to a plate.
- Distribute ¼ cup of the pimento cheese sauce over each slice of bread.
- Arrange half of the apple slices, caramelized onions, and arugula on top of each piece.
- Top each sandwich with a second slice of bread.
- Toast the first sandwich in the same pan you used for the onions for about two minutes, or over medium heat on a griddle, until the bottom slice of bread is golden brown.
- Using a silicone spatula, carefully flip the sandwich and cook for a further two minutes, or until the other side is browned.
- Move to a platter, then do the same with the other sandwich.
- Savor it warm.

NUTRITION FACTS:

- CALORIES: 465
- PROTEIN: 23g
- CARBS: 56g
- FAT: 10g

Apple Chickpea Salad Sandwich

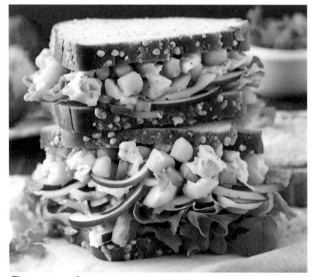

Serves: 1

Ingredients:

- 1 (15-ounce) can chickpeas, drained and rinsed
- ½ cup plain, unsweetened coconut yogurt
- ½ cup diced Fuji apple
- ⅓ cup finely diced celery
- ⅓ cup finely diced red onion
- 1 teaspoon fresh lemon juice
- ½ teaspoon garlic salt
- 3 drops of stevia or monk fruit sweetener
- Freshly ground black pepper, to taste
- 8 slices sprouted whole-grain

bread

- 8 romaine lettuce leaves 1 cup sprouts

Directions:

- Mash the chickpeas in a medium-sized bowl using a fork or potato masher. (It's okay if they seem a little chunky.)
- Incorporate the yogurt, apple, celery, onion, lemon juice, stevia, garlic salt, and a few of black pepper twists. Toss to combine well.
- Place a ½ cup of the filling on top of each of the four bread slices.
- Top each sandwich with two lettuce leaves and ¼ cup of sprouts.
- Place the second piece of bread on top of each sandwich and serve.

NUTRITION FACTS:

- CALORIES: 286
- PROTEIN: 14g
- CARBS: 39g
- FAT: 4g

Saucy Portobello Sammies

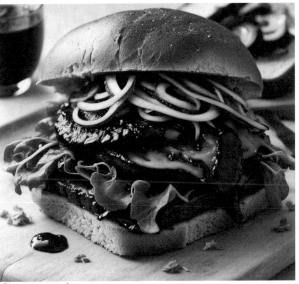

Serves: 1

Ingredients:

- Cooking spray (optional)
- 8 ounces portobello mushrooms, wiped clean, stems removed, and sliced
- 2 tablespoons of your favorite barbecue sauce (ideally one around 70 calories or fewer for 2 tablespoons)
- 2 slices sprouted whole-grain bread (see page 33)
- 2 tablespoons Smokehouse Ranch
- 2 slices red onion 1 cup spring greens
- ½ cup alfalfa sprouts

Directions:

- Turn up the heat to medium-high in a large nonstick skillet.
- You can use cooking spray to brown the mushrooms, but it's

- optional.
- Add the sliced mushrooms and simmer for about 8 minutes, stirring now and again, until they start to soften and brown.
- Sprinkle in a little water if the mushrooms start to stick. Take off the pan's heat source.
- Place the mushrooms and barbecue sauce in a small bowl, tossing to coat.
- Place the mushrooms, ranch, onion, greens, and sprouts on top of one slice of bread.
- Place the second piece of bread on top, then savor.

NUTRITION FACTS:
- CALORIES: 322
- PROTEIN: 13g
- CARBS: 46g
- FAT: 6g

Grilled Steak and Cheese Sammy

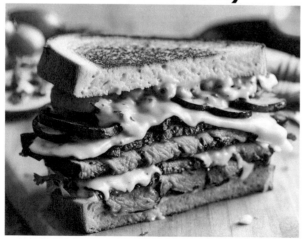

Serves: 1
Ingredients:
- Cooking spray (optional)
- 1 portobello mushroom cap (110g), wiped clean and thinly sliced
- ½ small yellow onion, thinly sliced
- Garlic salt, to taste
- ½cup Poblano Cheese Sauce, cold
- 2 slices of sprouted grain bread

Directions:
- Turn up the heat to medium-high in a large nonstick skillet.
- You can use cooking spray to ensure consistent cooking, but it's optional.
- Add the onion and mushroom, along with a dash of garlic salt, and sauté for about 8 minutes, or until the veggies are tender.
- If they begin to stick, add a splash of water. Take the pan off the heat.
- Drizzle one slice of bread with Poblano Cheese Sauce. Put the mushroom and onion mixture on top of the cheese, then the second layer of bread.
- Give your nonstick skillet a thorough cleaning, give it a

- quick spritz of cooking spray and put it back on medium heat.
- After adding the sandwich, grill it for about three minutes, or until the first side is golden brown. Flip the sandwich carefully, then continue on the other side.
- Serve warm.

NUTRITION FACTS:
- CALORIES: 268
- PROTEIN: 12g
- CARBS: 38g
- FAT: 5g

Hawaiian Street Cart Tacos

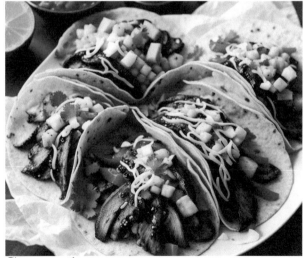

Serves: 1

Ingredients:
- Cooking spray (optional)
- 8 ounces portobello mushrooms, wiped clean, stems removed, and chopped
- ¼ teaspoon garlic salt
- 2 tablespoons of your favorite sweet barbecue sauce
- 4 (6-inch) corn tortillas
- ½ cup diced canned or fresh pineapple
- ¼ cup diced red bell pepper
- 1 scallion, sliced (white and green parts)
- Lime, for serving
- 2 tablespoons Smokehouse Ranch
- Chopped fresh cilantro leaves, for garnish

Directions:
- Turn up the heat to medium-high in a large nonstick pan.
- You can use cooking spray to ensure consistent cooking, but it's optional.
- After adding the mushrooms, season with the salt from garlic.
- Cook for 5 to 8 minutes, or until the mushrooms start to soften and become brown. Add a spritz of water if they begin to stick.
- Combine the mushrooms and barbecue sauce in a small bowl. Put aside.
- Clean the pan and spray it with

a thin layer of cooking spray.

- Set the skillet over medium heat and, one by one, reheat the tortillas for one to two minutes on each side, or just long enough to cook off the raw corn flavor.
- Distribute the filling of mushrooms among the tortillas.
- Add the scallion, bell pepper, and pineapple on top.
- Squeeze in some lime juice, then pour Smokehouse Ranch over the top. After adding the cilantro, serve.

NUTRITION FACTS:

- CALORIES: 372
- PROTEIN: 9g
- CARBS: 69g
- FAT: 4g

Loaded Taco Sweet Potato

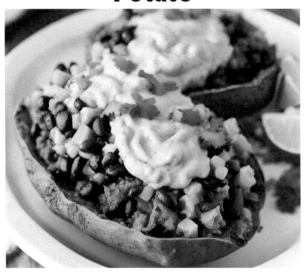

Serves: 1

Ingredients:

- 1 medium sweet potato (280g)
- ¼ cup (43g) canned black beans, drained and rinsed
- ¼ cup (41g) fresh or canned corn (drained, if canned)
- 2 tablespoons Summer Guac
- ¼ cup Poblano Cheese Sauce, warmed
- 2 tablespoons Cashew Lime Crema
- ¼ cup Pico de Gallo

Directions:

- Set the oven's temperature to 425°F. Place parchment paper on a baking pan and set it aside.
- Using a knife, pierce the sweet potato all over.
- Place it on the baking sheet that has been prepared, and bake for 45 to 60 minutes, or until a knife easily goes into the centre.
- Slice the sweet potato in half lengthwise and use a fork to fluff the centre once it is cold enough to handle.
- Place the beans, corn and Summer Guac on top of each half, and then pour the Cashew Lime Crema and Poblano

Cheese Sauce over them.

- Add a dollop of Pico de Gallo over top and enjoy.

NUTRITION FACTS:
- CALORIES: 529
- PROTEIN: 16g
- CARBS: 74g
- FAT: 14g

Spinach and Artichoke–Stuffed Mushrooms

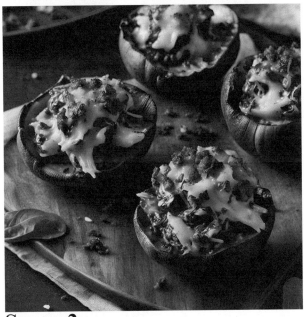

Serves: 2

Ingredients:
- 5 large portobello mushroom caps (400g), wiped clean
- Cooking spray (optional)
- 1 teaspoon garlic salt, divided
- ½ teaspoon smoked paprika
- 2 medium russet potatoes (426g), peeled and cubed
- 1 cup baby spinach leaves
- ¼ cup plain, unsweetened almond milk
- ½ cup canned artichoke hearts in water, drained
- 1¼ cups Garlic Alfredo Sauce, warmed

Directions:
- Set the oven's temperature to 375°F. Place parchment paper on a baking pan and set it aside.
- Lightly moisten the mushrooms all over with water using your fingers, or lightly coat them with cooking spray. (This is merely to prevent the mushrooms from drying out in the oven and to aid in the seasonings sticking.)
- Season the mushrooms, top and bottom, with ½ teaspoon garlic salt and smoked paprika.
- Place them face down on the baking sheet. Bake for fifteen minutes. Put aside.
- In the meantime, place the potatoes in a medium-sized saucepan and fill it with just enough water to cover them.
- Over medium-high heat, bring to a boil, then lower the heat to a simmer and cook for about 15

minutes, or until the potatoes are fork tender.

- After transferring them to a medium-sized bowl, let them cool slightly.
- Steam the spinach while the potatoes and mushrooms are cooking.
- Fill a medium saucepan with 2 inches of water and insert a steamer basket.
- Over medium heat, bring the water to a simmer, add the spinach, cover, and steam for about two minutes, or until the spinach is bright green and just tender.
- Move to a bowl or platter, then put it aside.
- After the potatoes have cooled down a little, mash them largely smooth using a fork or potato masher.
- Mix thoroughly after adding the almond milk and the remaining ½ teaspoon of garlic salt.
- Add spinach and artichoke hearts and toss until equally distributed.
- Add ½ cup mashed potatoes and ¼ cup Garlic Alfredo

Sauce to each mushroom.
- Serve warm.

NUTRITION FACTS:
- CALORIES: 312
- PROTEIN: 12g
- CARBS: 49g
- FAT: 5g

Yellow Potato Curry

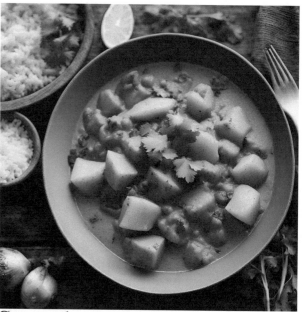

Serves: 1

Ingredients:
- ½ cup diced yellow onion
- 2 teaspoons curry powder
- 2 teaspoons minced garlic
- 2 teaspoons minced ginger
- 1 teaspoon garam masala
- ¼ teaspoon turmeric powder
- ¾ teaspoon sea salt, plus more to taste
- ½ cup water
- 2 cups plain, unsweetened

- almond milk
- 1 large Yukon Gold potato (425g), cubed but not peeled
- ½ cup frozen peas
- Stevia, to taste
- Lime, for serving
- 1 tablespoon chopped fresh cilantro leaves
- 1 cup cooked (158g) white or brown rice, for serving (optional)

Directions:

- Combine the onion, curry powder, garlic, ginger, garam masala, turmeric, and salt in a medium-sized pot over medium heat.
- Cook for about five minutes, or until the onions are transparent and the spices are fragrant, after adding the water.
- Add almond milk and potatoes, then boil for 15 minutes or until fork tender.
- Remove from heat and stir in peas to defrost.
- Taste and add additional salt, lime juice, and a few drops of stevia, if necessary.
- Add cilantro as a garnish and, if preferred, pair with rice.

NUTRITION FACTS:

- CALORIES: 463
- PROTEIN: 11g
- CARBS: 88g
- FAT: 4g

Cauliflower Steak Dinner with Mashed Potatoes and Green Beans

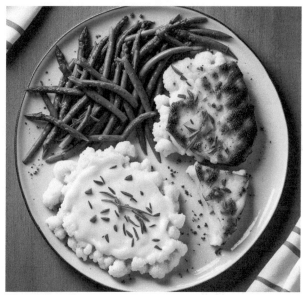

Serves: 1

Ingredients:

For The Steaks

- 1 medium head of cauliflower
- Cooking spray (see page 33)
- Garlic salt and freshly ground black pepper, to taste

For The Mashed Potatoes

- 1 large Yukon gold potato (350g)
- ¼ cup plain, unsweetened almond milk

- ½ teaspoon garlic salt, plus more to taste
- 1 teaspoon chopped chives, for garnish

For The Greens Beans
- 3½ cups fresh or frozen green beans, ends trimmed
- ⅛ teaspoon garlic salt
- Lemon, for serving
- 1 tablespoon vegan
- Worcestershire or steak sauce, for serving (optional)

Directions:
- Start by preheating the oven to 425°F for the steaks.
- Cut the stem off of the cauliflower at its base. Place the cauliflower on its flat side and cut three steaks that are one inch thick.
- The leftover cauliflower can be cooked and frozen for a later dinner, or it can be kept raw and used to make Falafel Cauliflower Pitas.
- Use parchment paper to line a baking sheet.
- Place cauliflower slices on a sheet pan and lightly spray both sides with cooking spray to brown and prevent drying. Garlic salt and pepper should be used to season both sides.
- Roast for 30 minutes, turning halfway through, or until the edges are crispy and golden brown.
- In the meantime, prepare the mashed potatoes by putting them in a medium pot with just enough cold water to cover them.
- Over medium-high heat, bring to a boil and then lower the heat to a simmer.
- Simmer for about 15 minutes, or until the potatoes are fork-tender.
- Move the potatoes to a medium-sized bowl and mash them with a fork or potato masher.
- Stir in the garlic salt and almond milk. Season with extra garlic salt if preferred, then sprinkle with chives and set aside.
- Prepare the green beans by filling a medium saucepan with one inch of water while the potatoes are boiling.
- Place a steamer basket inside the pot and heat it to a medium simmer. Put the green beans in

the steamer basket, cover it, and steam for three to five minutes, or until they are bright green and somewhat soft.

- Move the green beans into a medium-sized bowl and mix with the garlic salt. Add a squeeze of lemon to finish.
- If preferred, serve the steaks with Worcestershire or steak sauce for dipping along with the mashed potatoes and green beans.

NUTRITION FACTS:
- CALORIES: 534
- PROTEIN: 24g
- CARBS: 88g
- FAT: 3g

Cauliflower Masala

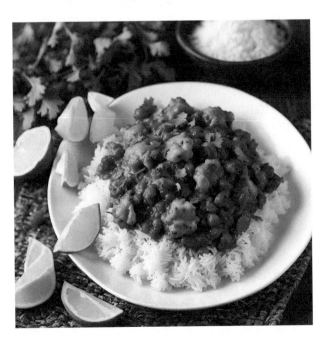

Serves: 2

Ingredients:
- 1 (14.5-ounce) can diced tomatoes
- ½ medium yellow onion
- 2 teaspoons minced garlic
- 1 teaspoon minced ginger or ¼ teaspoon dried ginger
- 1½ teaspoons tikka masala powder
- 1½ teaspoons curry powder
- 1 teaspoon sea salt, or more to taste
- 1 medium head of cauliflower, stemmed and chopped (about 7 cups or 650g)
- 2 cups unsweetened almond milk
- ¼ cup chopped fresh cilantro leaves
- Stevia, to taste
- Lime, for serving
- 2 cups (316g) cooked white or brown rice, for serving (optional)

Directions:
- Put the tomatoes, onion, garlic, and ginger in a blender and process until smooth.
- Move to a big saucepan that is heated to a medium-high temperature. Stir in the curry

powder, tikka masala powder, and salt. Simmer for 4 minutes, or until the sauce begins to slightly thicken, stirring occasionally.

- Add the cauliflower and almond milk, and cook for 10 to 12 minutes, or until the cauliflower is soft.
- Take the pot off of the heat and add the stevia, lime juice and cilantro.
- The meal should have a mild, sweet flavour.
- If necessary, add extra salt to the seasoning and serve over rice.

NUTRITION FACTS:
- CALORIES: 614
- PROTEIN: 19g
- CARBS: 111g
- FAT: 5g

Vegan Crab Cakes

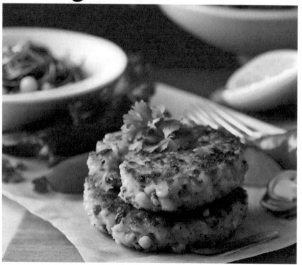

Serves: 2

Ingredients:
- 1 (15-ounce) can chickpeas, drained and rinsed
- 1 (14-ounce) can hearts of palm packed in water, drained
- ⅓ cup minced red onion
- ⅓ cup minced red bell pepper
- ¼ cup chopped fresh parsley leaves
- 1 tablespoon Dijon mustard
- 1 tablespoon brined capers, drained
- 2½ teaspoons Old Bay seasoning
- 1 teaspoon fresh lemon juice
- 1 teaspoon chopped fresh dill
- ½ teaspoon kelp granules
- ½ cup panko breadcrumbs
- Cooking spray (optional)
- Remoulade, for serving (optional)

Directions:
- Place the chickpeas, lemon juice, dill, kelp granules, onion, bell pepper, parsley, Dijon, capers, Old Bay, and hearts of palm in the bowl of a food processor. Pulse the chickpeas until they break up thoroughly. Fold in breadcrumbs evenly using a spatula.

- Using your hands, shape a loose ½ cup of the filling into a patty that is ½ inch thick.
- Turn up the heat to medium in a large nonstick skillet. You can use cooking spray to ensure consistent cooking, but it's optional.
- Add patties in batches to avoid overcrowding the pan.
- After about three minutes, or when the first side is golden brown, turn it over and continue on the second side.
- If preferred, serve with the Remoulade.

NUTRITION FACTS:
- CALORIES: 397
- PROTEIN: 18g
- CARBS: 46g
- FAT: 12g

Cilantro-Lime Stuffed Peppers

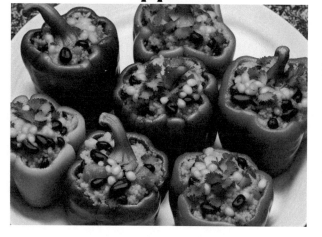

Serves: 1

Ingredients:
- 3 large bell peppers (any color)
- 1 cup (159g) cooked white or brown rice
- ¼ cup (43g) canned black beans, drained and rinsed
- ¼ cup (41g) fresh or canned corn (drained, if canned)
- 3 tablespoons store-bought or homemade salsa
- 2 tablespoons chopped fresh cilantro leaves
- 1 teaspoon fresh lime juice
- Garlic salt, to taste
- ¾ cup Poblano Cheese Sauce, warmed

Directions:
- Set the oven's temperature to 425°F. Use parchment paper to line a baking sheet, then set it aside.
- Cut off the tops of the bell peppers, then remove the seeds and ribs with a spoon. Place the peppers on a separate plate.
- Combine the rice, beans, corn, salsa, cilantro and lime juice in a medium-sized bowl. Use the garlic salt to season to taste.
- Divide the filling evenly among the peppers and place them on

the baking sheet. After roasting for 25 minutes, the peppers should be tender and starting to colour.

- Drizzle the Poblano Cheese Sauce over the peppers and serve.

NUTRITION FACTS:
- CALORIES: 563
- PROTEIN: 18g
- CARBS: 93g
- FAT: 8g

Cheesy Poblano Enchiladas

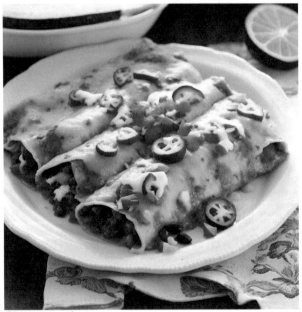

Serves: 1

Ingredients:
- Cooking spray (optional)
- 1 medium zucchini, diced (about 2 cups)
- 1 red bell pepper, seeded and diced (1 cup)
- ¾ cup diced yellow onion
- ¾ cup low-fat or fat-free green enchilada sauce
- ½ cup (86g) canned pinto beans, drained and rinsed
- ¼ cup (41g) fresh or canned corn (drained, if canned)
- ⅓ cup chopped fresh cilantro leaves 4 (10-inch) flour tortillas
- ½ cup Poblano Cheese Sauce
- ¼ small avocado (25g), for serving (optional)
- Cashew Lime Crema, for serving (optional)

Directions:
- Set oven temperature to 375°F.
- Turn up the heat to medium-high in a large nonstick skillet. You can use cooking spray to ensure consistent cooking, but it's optional.
- Add the onion, bell pepper, and zucchini, and sauté for 8 to 10 minutes, or until the veggies are tender and starting to brown.
- You can add a splash of water if the vegetables begin to stick.
- Put the sautéed veggies, beans, corn, cilantro, and ½ cup of the enchilada sauce in a medium-sized bowl. Mix thoroughly by stirring.

- Spoon about 1/4 of the contents onto a tortilla that has been laid out on a surface.
- The tortilla should be rolled up and put in a 6 x 12 inch baking tray. Proceed with the leftover tortillas and filling.
- After adding the last ¼ cup of enchilada sauce to the enchiladas, bake them for 20 minutes, or until they are well heated.
- Add the avocado and/or cashew lime crema on top of the enchiladas, along with the Poblano Cheese Sauce, if preferred.

NUTRITION FACTS:
- CALORIES: 423
- PROTEIN: 27g
- CARBS: 88g
- FAT: 16g

Creamy Roasted Pepper Pasta

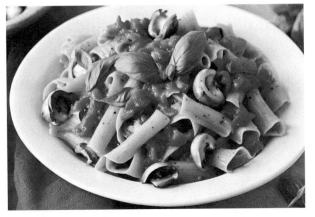

Serves: 1
Ingredients:
- 4 ounces uncooked whole-grain pasta
- Cooking spray (optional)
- 8 ounces baby bella mushrooms, wiped clean and quartered
- ½ cup Roasted Red Pepper Sauce
- 1 tablespoon chopped fresh basil leaves

Directions:
- Prepare the pasta per the directions on the package, drain, and transfer to a medium-sized bowl. Put aside.
- Turn up the heat to medium-high in a large nonstick skillet.
- You can use cooking spray to brown the mushrooms, but it's optional. Add the mushrooms and simmer for about 8 minutes, or until they are tender and starting to brown.
- Add a spritz of water if they begin to stick.
- Add the mushrooms to the pasta bowl. Pour the Roasted Red Pepper Sauce on top and mix to ensure a thorough coating.

- Garnish with chopped basil.

NUTRITION FACTS:
- CALORIES: 540
- PROTEIN: 25g
- CARBS: 89g
- FAT: 7g

Lean Lasagna

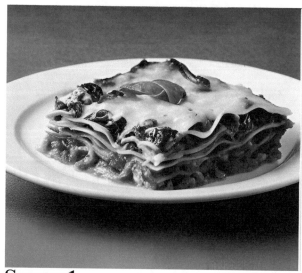

Serves: 1

Ingredients:
- Cooking spray (optional)
- 16 ounces white mushrooms, wiped clean and chopped
- ⅔ block (370g/100 oz) extra-firm tofu
- 2 cups packed fresh baby spinach leaves
- 1 cup (170g) canned artichoke hearts, drained and chopped
- ¼ cup nutritional yeast
- 2 tablespoons fresh lemon juice
- 1 teaspoon garlic salt, plus more to taste 1 teaspoon Italian seasoning
- ¼ teaspoon onion powder
- ¼ teaspoon garlic powder
- 3 cups fat-free marinara sauce
- 8 to 12 sheets no-bake lasagna noodles 288g (use gluten free, if desired)
- Grated vegan Parmesan, optional

Directions:
- Set the oven's temperature to 375°F.
- Turn up the heat to medium-high in a large nonstick skillet.
- You can use cooking spray to ensure consistent cooking, but it's optional.
- Add the mushrooms and sauté for about 6 minutes, or until they are tender. If they stick, add a spritz of water.
- Put the sautéed mushrooms, tofu, spinach, artichoke hearts, nutritional yeast, lemon juice, Italian seasoning, garlic salt, onion powder, and garlic powder in a food processor.
- The mixture should become smooth and creamy, akin to ricotta after a few pulses.
- Season with extra garlic salt if desired.

- In an 8 x 12-inch casserole dish, spread a tablespoon of marinara over the bottom.
- First place a layer of noodles, then cover it with ½ cup of the tofu mixture.
- Next, add a dollop of marinara and another layer of noodles.
- Keep layering until you run out of noodles, setting aside ½ cup of the marinara.
- Add ¼ cup water to the dish, cover with foil, and bake for 45-55 minutes until noodles are fully cooked.
- Let the lasagna cool a little before adding the final ½ cup of marinara and, if preferred, some vegan Parmesan.
- Cut into pieces and serve.

NUTRITION FACTS:
- CALORIES: 627
- PROTEIN: 47g
- CARBS: 75g
- FAT: 10g

Mushroom Stroganoff

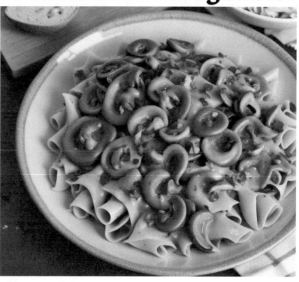

Serves: 2

Ingredients:
- 6 ounces uncooked pasta of your choice
- ½ cup plain, unsweetened almond milk
- ¼ cup raw cashews (130g)
- Cooking spray (optional)
- 8 ounces baby bella mushrooms, sliced or quartered
- ½ small yellow onion (110g), diced
- 2 tablespoons vegan Worcestershire sauce
- Garlic salt, to taste
- Ground black pepper, to taste
- 1 tablespoon chopped fresh parsley leaves, for garnish
- Grated plant-based Parmesan, for serving (optional)

Directions:

- Pour water into a medium pot and heat it to a boil over medium-high heat.
- Following the directions on the package, add the pasta and cook. Once drained, set aside.
- Begin the sauce while the pasta cooks. Almond milk and cashews should be combined in a blender and blended until smooth. Put aside.
- Turn up the heat to medium-high in a big nonstick skillet.
- You can use cooking spray to ensure consistent cooking, but it's optional.
- Add the onion and mushrooms, and sauté for 8 to 10 minutes, or until the vegetables have softened and started to brown.
- You can add a little water if they begin to stick.
- Take the pan off the heat and add the Worcestershire sauce and the cashew mixture.
- Incorporate the pasta and mix to thoroughly coat.
- Add pepper and garlic salt to taste, and then sprinkle the parsley on top.
- If preferred, top the dish with a little Parmesan cheese.

NUTRITION FACTS:
- CALORIES: 450
- PROTEIN: 19g
- CARBS: 67g
- FAT: 11g

Smoky Sweet Chili

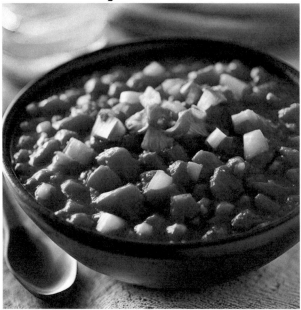

Serves: 2

Ingredients:
- 1 (15-ounce) can chili beans, drained
- 1 (14-ounce) can diced tomatoes
- ½ small yellow onion (110g), diced
- 1 tablespoon minced garlic
- 1 tablespoon ketchup
- 1 tablespoon maple syrup
- 1 to 2 teaspoons chipotle powder (depending on how much spice you like; optional)

- 1 teaspoon smoked paprika
- ½ teaspoon chili powder
- ¼ teaspoon garlic salt, plus more to taste
- Lime, for serving
- Chopped fresh cilantro, for serving
- 3 tablespoons Cashew Lime Crema

Directions:

- The beans, tomatoes, onion, garlic, ketchup, maple syrup, paprika, chili powder, garlic salt, and chipotle powder (if used) should all be combined in a medium-sized pot over medium-high heat.
- After bringing the mixture to a boil, lower the heat to a simmer, and continue cooking for five to ten minutes, or until well heated.
- Add extra garlic salt for seasoning, if necessary.
- Garnish with a lime wedge, cilantro sprigs, and a dab of cashew lime crema.

NUTRITION FACTS:

- CALORIES: 657
- PROTEIN: 26g
- CARBS: 88g
- FAT: 13g

Teriyaki Bowl

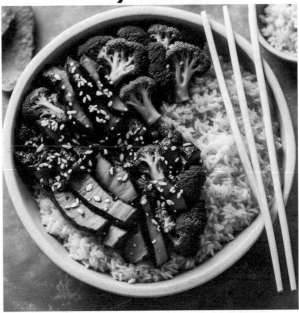

Serves: 1

Ingredients:

- 2 cups fresh or frozen broccoli florets
- Cooking spray (optional)
- 8 ounces portobello mushroom caps, wiped clean and sliced
- Pinch of garlic salt
- 2 cups (316g) white or brown rice, steamed
- 4 tablespoons Teriyaki Sauce
- ¼ teaspoon black sesame seeds

Directions:

- Simmer two inches of water in a medium saucepan with a fitting lid.
- Put the steamer basket in the pot with the broccoli inside of it.

- For five minutes, with the pot covered, steam the broccoli until it turns bright green and becomes somewhat soft but not mushy.
- As an alternative, you can put the broccoli in a microwave-safe container, cover it, and cook it in the microwave for four minutes. Put aside.
- Turn up the heat to medium in a large nonstick skillet. Spraying the pan with cooking spray can help brown the mushrooms, but it's optional.
- Add the mushrooms and sprinkle the garlic salt over them. Cook for 5 to 8 minutes, or until the mushrooms are soft.
- A quick spray of water can be added if the mushrooms begin to stick. Take the pan off heat.
- Make a bed of rice in a serving bowl, then add the broccoli and mushrooms on top.
- After adding the sesame seeds, drizzle with the Teriyaki sauce and serve.

NUTRITION FACTS:
- CALORIES: 548
- PROTEIN: 17g
- CARBS: 109g
- FAT: 3g

Fajita Bowl

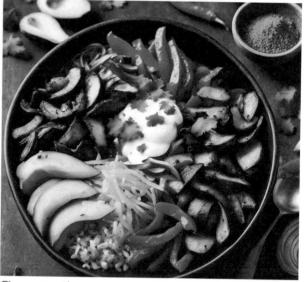

Serves: 1

Ingredients:
- 1 medium Yukon gold potato (325g)
- 1 red bell pepper, seeded and sliced
- 1 small red onion (150g), sliced
- 1 portobello mushroom cap (110g), sliced
- ½ teaspoon chili powder or fajita/taco seasoning
- Smoked paprika, to taste
- Garlic salt, to taste
- 4 cups (80g) spring greens
- ¼ medium avocado (25g), optional
- ½ cup Smokehouse Ranch
- ¼ cup chopped fresh cilantro, for garnish, optional

Directions:

- Transfer the potato to a small pot and cover with just enough water. The water should be brought to a boil over medium-high heat and then reduced to a simmer.
- Simmer the potato for about 20 minutes, or until it is fork-tender. After draining, place somewhere to cool slightly.
- Dice the potato into 1-inch pieces once it has cooled enough to handle.
- Set oven temperature to 375°F.
- Spread parchment paper on a baking sheet and arrange the chopped onion, bell pepper, potato, and mushroom.
- Add a dash of smoky paprika, garlic salt, and chili powder for seasoning.
- After giving the veggies a good toss, distribute them evenly around the sheet.
- Roast the vegetables for 15 to 20 minutes, or until they are soft and starting to turn brown.
- Transfer the roasted veggies to a large bowl and mix with the greens.
- Arrange the avocado (if using),

- Smokehouse Ranch, cilantro, and hot sauce (if like) on top.

NUTRITION FACTS:

- CALORIES: 562
- PROTEIN: 18g
- CARBS: 75g
- FAT: 19g

Chickpea Avocado Bowl

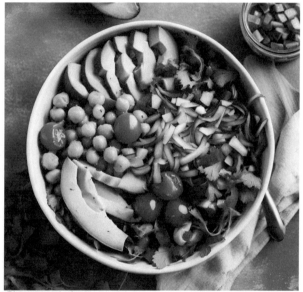

Serves: 1

Ingredients:

- 4 cups spring greens
- ½ cup cherry tomatoes, halved
- ½ cup sliced English cucumber
- 1 cup canned chickpeas (164g), drained and rinsed
- ½ medium avocado (50g), peeled, pitted, and sliced
- ¼ cup red onion (from 1 small onion)
- ¼ cup fresh cilantro leaves, chopped

- 6 tablespoons Lemon-Herb Caesar

Directions:

- Combine the greens, avocado, onion, cucumber, chickpeas, tomatoes, and cilantro in a medium-sized bowl.
- Pour over the dressing and toss once more to mix.

NUTRITION FACTS:

- CALORIES: 185
- PROTEIN: 23g
- CARBS: 46g
- FAT: 22g

Japanese Nourish Bowl

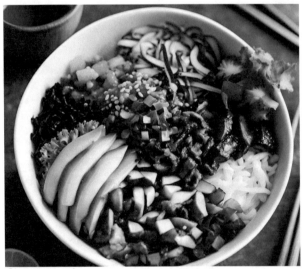

Serves: 1

Ingredients:

- Cooking spray (optional)
- 5 ounces shiitake mushrooms, wiped clean, stems removed, and sliced
- ½ small yellow onion (110g), diced
- 3 tablespoons teriyaki coconut aminos
- 1 tablespoon minced garlic
- 1 teaspoon oil-free chili paste (I like sambal oelek)
- ½ teaspoon minced fresh ginger
- 2 cups chopped kale leaves
- 1 ½ cups (237g) cooked white or brown rice Chopped scallions (green parts only), for serving
- ¼ teaspoon sesame oil Sesame seeds, for serving
- Teriyaki seaweed, for serving (optional)

Directions:

- Turn up the heat to medium in a large nonstick skillet.
- Coating the pan with cooking spray can help ensure consistent cooking, but it's optional.
- Add the onion, mushrooms, and teriyaki coconut aminos. Cook, stirring often, for about 5 minutes, or until the onion and mushrooms are soft.
- You can add a splash of water if the vegetables begin to stick.
- Add the ginger, garlic, and chili paste. Cook, stirring, for

about two minutes, or until aromatic.

- Add the kale and simmer, stirring, for about 2 minutes, or until wilted and tender. Take the pan off of the heat.
- In a medium-sized serving bowl, add the rice and then the kale mixture on top.
- If preferred, serve with teriyaki seaweed and garnish with sesame oil, sesame seeds, and scallions.

NUTRITION FACTS:
- CALORIES: 443
- PROTEIN: 12g
- CARBS: 80g
- FAT: 5g

Butternut Squash and Kale Salad with Cranberries and Pecans

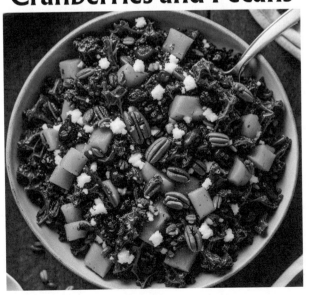

Serves: 1

Ingredients:
- 2 cups peeled and cubed butternut squash
- Cooking spray
- ¼ teaspoon garlic salt
- Freshly ground black pepper, to taste
- 1 cup water
- ¼ cup dry white quinoa (170g)
- 3 cups shredded lacinato kale leaves
- 2 tablespoons dried cranberries
- 1 tablespoon pecans, toasted in a dry pan until fragrant
- ¼ cup Lemon-Herb Caesar dressing

Directions:
- Set the oven's temperature to 425°F. Put parchment paper on a baking pan.
- Place the squash on the baking sheet and spray it with cooking spray just a little bit.
- Apply a small amount of pepper and garlic salt for seasoning, then spread into a single, equal layer. Bake for about 20 minutes, or until starting to brown.
- In the meantime, fill a medium saucepan with water and raise it

to a boil over medium-high heat. Reduce to a simmer after adding the quinoa.

- As directed by the package, cook, covered, for approximately 15 minutes, or until all of the water has been absorbed. Take the pot off of the heat.
- To a large bowl, add the kale, pecans, and cranberries.
- Add the squash and quinoa on top, pour the lemon-herb Caesar dressing over it, and toss to mix

NUTRITION FACTS:
- CALORIES: 482
- PROTEIN: 14g
- CARBS: 65g
- FAT: 16g

Sauces, Dressings and Dips

All-Purpose Asian Dressing

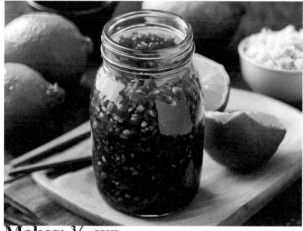

Makes: ¾ cup

Ingredients:

- ¼ cup low-sodium soy sauce
- 3 tablespoons fresh lime juice
- 3 tablespoons water
- 1 small shallot, minced
- 2 teaspoons chili paste
- 1 teaspoon minced garlic
- ½ teaspoon toasted sesame oil
- ½ teaspoon minced ginger or ¼ teaspoon ground ginger
- Pinch of chili flakes
- 3 to 4 drops of stevia or monk fruit sweetener

Directions:

- Combine the soy sauce, lime juice, water, sesame oil, ginger, shallot, chili paste, and garlic in a medium-sized bowl.
- Use stevia or monk fruit sweetener to taste-test and adjust the flavor.
- For up to five days, keep in the refrigerator in a tightly closed jar or container.

NUTRITION FACTS FOR 1 TB:

- CALORIES: 7
- PROTEIN: 1g
- CARBS: 1g
- FAT: 0g

Creamy Sriracha Dressing

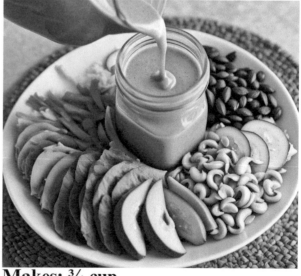

Makes: ¾ cup

Ingredients:

- ½ cup raw cashews
- ½ cup plain, unsweetened

almond milk

- 1 tablespoon sriracha, plus more to taste
- 1 teaspoon rice vinegar
- ½ teaspoon sea salt
- ¼ teaspoon garlic powder
- ⅛ teaspoon toasted sesame oil

Directions:

- Combine the soy sauce, lime juice, water, sesame oil, ginger, shallot, chili paste, and garlic in

Pesto Dressing

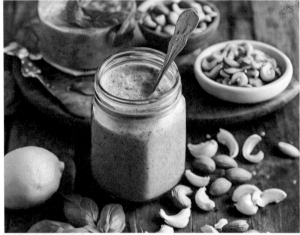

Makes: ⅔ cup

Ingredients:

- ½ cup plain, unsweetened almond milk
- ½ cup packed fresh basil
- 2 tablespoons raw cashews
- 1 tablespoon fresh lemon juice
- ¼ teaspoon garlic powder
- ⅛ teaspoon sea salt, plus more to taste

Directions:

- Put the almond milk, cashews, basil, lemon juice, garlic powder, and salt in a blender.
- Process until smooth, then adjust the seasoning with additional salt if needed.
- For up to five days, keep in the refrigerator in a tightly closed jar or container.

NUTRITION FACTS:

- CALORIES: 60
- PROTEIN: 2g
- CARBS: 3g
- FAT: 4g

Smokehouse Ranch

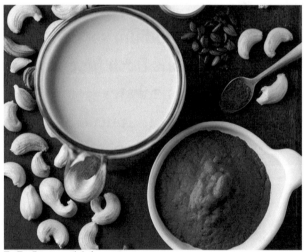

Makes: 1⅓ cup

Ingredients:

- 1 cup plain, unsweetened almond milk
- ¾ cup raw cashews
- 1 tablespoon distilled white vinegar
- 1 tablespoon ketchup

- ½ teaspoon smoked paprika
- ¼ teaspoon garlic powder
- ⅛ teaspoon onion powder
- ⅛ teaspoon chipotle powder
- 3 drops stevia sweetener
- 1 tablespoon dried chives
- 1 tablespoon dried parsley

Directions:

- The almond milk, cashews, vinegar, ketchup, smoked paprika, onion, garlic, chipotle, and stevia should all be combined in a blender.
- Process till smooth. Add the parsley and chives and fold them in with a spoon or spatula.
- For up to five days, keep in the refrigerator in a sealed container.

NUTRITION FACTS:

- CALORIES: 27
- PROTEIN: 1g
- CARBS: 2g
- FAT: 2g

Lemon-Herb Caesar

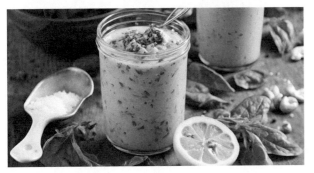

Makes: 1¾ cup

Ingredients:

- 1 cup plain, unsweetened almond milk
- ¾ cup raw cashews
- 2 tablespoons fresh lemon juice
- 2 teaspoons brine-packed capers, drained, plus
- 3 teaspoons caper brine
- 2 teaspoons Dijon mustard
- ½ teaspoon sea salt, plus more to taste
- ¼ teaspoon garlic powder
- ⅛ teaspoon onion powder
- Freshly ground black pepper, to taste
- 2 tablespoons dried chives
- 1 tablespoon dried parsley

Directions:

- Almond milk, cashews, lemon juice, brine and capers, Dijon, salt, onion and garlic powder, and a few grinds of black pepper should all be combined in a blender.
- Process till smooth. Fold in the herbs with a spoon or spatula, and add additional salt and pepper to taste.
- For up to five days, keep in the refrigerator in a sealed container.

NUTRITION FACTS:
- CALORIES: 22
- PROTEIN: 1g
- CARBS: 1g
- FAT: 2g

Simple Hummus

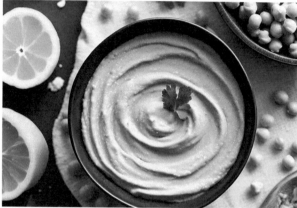

Makes: 1 cup

Ingredients:

- 1 (15-ounce) can chickpeas, drained and rinsed
- ¼ cup water
- 1 tablespoon fresh lemon juice
- ½ tablespoon tahini paste
- ½ teaspoon sea salt
- ¼ teaspoon garlic powder
- ⅛ teaspoon ground cumin

Directions:

- Put the chickpeas, water, lemon juice, tahini paste, cumin, salt, and garlic powder in a blender.
- Process till smooth.
- For up to one week, keep in the refrigerator in a sealed container.

NUTRITION FACTS:
- CALORIES: 99
- PROTEIN: 5g
- CARBS: 10g
- FAT: 3g

Corn and Cucumber Salsa

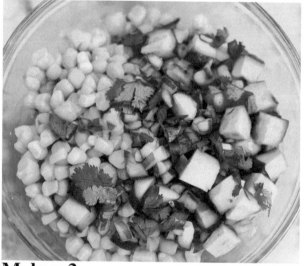

Makes: 3 cup

Ingredients:

- 1 (15-ounce) can corn, drained
- 1 cup diced English cucumber
- ½ medium avocado (55g), diced
- ¼ cup chopped red onion
- ¼ cup chopped fresh cilantro leaves
- Juice of 1 lime
- ¼ teaspoon sea salt, plus more to taste
- ⅛ teaspoon garlic powder

Directions:

- Combine the corn, avocado, cucumber, onion, cilantro, lime juice, salt, and garlic powder in a medium-sized bowl.

- Toss everything gently, and if needed, add more salt to taste.
- For up to four days, keep in the refrigerator in a sealed container.

NUTRITION FACTS:

- CALORIES: 52
- PROTEIN: 1g
- CARBS: 7g
- FAT: 2g

Pico de Gallo

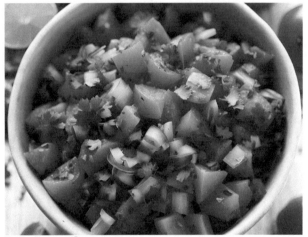

Makes: 2 cup

Ingredients:

- 1½ cups diced Roma tomatoes (about 3 medium tomatoes)
- ⅓ cup chopped fresh cilantro leaves ¼ cup diced red onion
- 2 tablespoons fresh lime juice
- ⅛ teaspoon sea salt, plus more to taste

Directions:

- Combine the tomatoes, onion, cilantro, lime juice, and salt in a medium-sized bowl.
- Toss everything gently, and if needed, add more salt to taste.
- For up to four days, keep in the refrigerator in a sealed container.

NUTRITION FACTS:

- CALORIES: 21
- PROTEIN: 1g
- CARBS: 4g
- FAT: 0g

Summer Guac

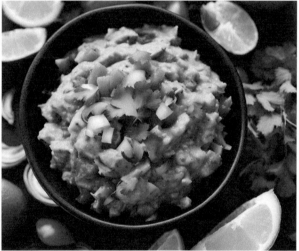

Makes: 1¼ cup

Ingredients:

- 2 medium avocados (210g), pitted and peeled
- ¼ cup diced Roma tomato (about 1 medium tomato)
- ¼ cup chopped fresh cilantro leaves
- 2 tablespoons minced red onion

- 2 tablespoons diced jalapeño
- 2 tablespoons fresh lime juice
- ¼ teaspoon sea salt, plus more to taste

Directions:
- Mash the avocado using a fork in a medium-sized bowl, adding as much chunks or smoothness as desired.
- Add the lime juice, salt, onion, jalapeño, tomato, and cilantro.
- Mix everything together gently, and if needed, add extra salt to taste.
- Keep refrigerated for up to 4 days in a sealed container.

NUTRITION FACTS:
- CALORIES: 82
- PROTEIN: 1g
- CARBS: 3g
- FAT: 7g

Teriyaki Sauce

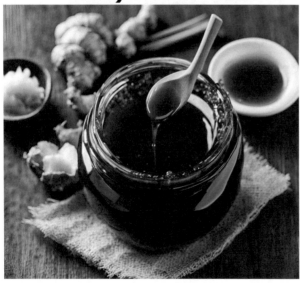

Makes: 1⅓ cup

Ingredients:
- 2 tablespoons corn-starch
- ½ cup low-sodium soy sauce
- ½ cup water
- ½ teaspoon minced garlic or ¼ teaspoon garlic powder
- ¼ teaspoon minced fresh ginger or ⅛ teaspoon powdered ginger
- ¼ cup maple syrup

Directions:
- Combine the corn-starch and ¼ cup of cold water in a small bowl. Put aside.
- Put the water, ginger, garlic, and soy sauce in a medium-sized pot.
- Over medium-high heat, bring the mixture to a simmer while stirring from time to time.
- Add the corn-starch mixture and stir for a further minute or so, or until the sauce thickens. Remove from heat and incorporate maple syrup.
- You may keep the sauce in the fridge for up to a week by storing it in a sealed jar or container.

NUTRITION FACTS:
- CALORIES: 17
- PROTEIN: 1g

- CARBS: 4g
- FAT: 0g

Poblano Cheese Sauce

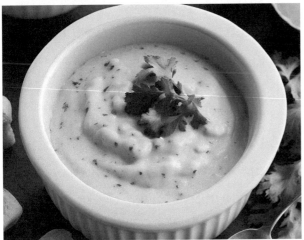

Makes: 2¼ cup

Ingredients:

- 1 medium poblano pepper
- 1½ cups (225g) peeled and diced Russet potatoes
- ¼ cup raw cashews
- 1 teaspoon fresh lemon juice
- 1 teaspoon garlic powder
- 1 teaspoon sea salt
- ½ teaspoon onion powder

Directions:

- Set the oven's temperature to 425°F. Put parchment paper on a baking pan.
- Arrange the poblano pepper on the baking sheet that has been prepared, and roast it for 20 minutes, or until it is nicely roasted all over.
- Meanwhile, prepare the potatoes. Add enough cold water to cover the potatoes by two inches in a small pot.
- Heat to a boil over medium-high heat, then lower the heat to a simmer and cook, uncovered, for 15 minutes or until the potatoes are soft.
- Drain the potatoes in a strainer and set aside, reserving 1 cup of the cooking water.
- As soon as the pepper is done roasting, move it to a bowl covered with plastic wrap or a plastic zip-top bag and steam it for ten minutes.
- Take the pepper out and let it to cool.
- Using your hands, remove the peel and remove the seeds after they are safe to handle (unless you want your sauce to be quite spicy!).
- Fill a blender with the pepper, cooked potatoes, and cooking water. Then, add the cashews, lemon juice, onion powder, garlic powder, and salt. Process till smooth.
- For up to a week, keep in the refrigerator in a sealed container.

- To reheat, place in the microwave and stir every 30 seconds or until the food is heated to your desired temperature.

NUTRITION FACTS:
- CALORIES: 43
- PROTEIN: 1g
- CARBS: 5g
- FAT: 2g

Avocado Lime Crema

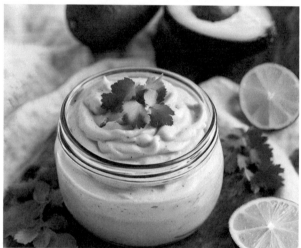

Makes: 2¼ cup

Ingredients:
- 2 medium avocados (250g), pitted, peeled, and scooped
- ½ cup chopped fresh cilantro leaves
- ½ cup water
- 1 medium jalapeño, seeds removed if you prefer less heat
- 5 tablespoons fresh lime juice (from about 2 large limes)
- ¼ teaspoon sea salt

- ¼ teaspoon garlic powder
- ¼ teaspoon onion powder

Directions:
- Put the avocados, cilantro, lime juice, jalapeño, water, salt, garlic powder, and onion powder in a blender. Process till smooth.
- For up to three days, keep in the refrigerator in a sealed container.

NUTRITION FACTS:
- CALORIES: 13
- PROTEIN: 0g
- CARBS: 1g
- FAT: 1g

Cashew Lime Crema

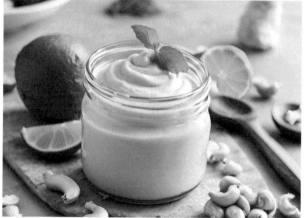

Makes: 2¼ cup

Ingredients:
- ¾ cup raw cashews, soaked overnight or boiled for 8 minutes
- ¼ cup water
- 5 teaspoons fresh lime juice

- 1½ teaspoons white vinegar
- ¼ teaspoon sea salt, plus more to taste
- ⅛ teaspoon garlic powder
- 2 drops of stevia sweetener

Directions:
- Put the cashews, water, vinegar, lime juice, salt, stevia, and garlic powder in a blender.
- Process till smooth. If preferred, season with more salt.
- For up to five days, keep in the refrigerator in a sealed container.

NUTRITION FACTS:
- CALORIES: 39
- PROTEIN: 1g
- CARBS: 2g
- FAT: 3g

Tzatziki Sauce

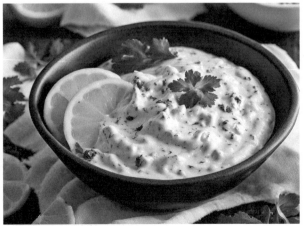

Makes: 1¼ cup
Ingredients:
- 1 cup plain unsweetened coconut yogurt
- ¼ cup chopped fresh parsley leaves
- 1 tablespoon fresh lemon juice
- ½ teaspoon minced garlic
- ¼ teaspoon sea salt, plus more to taste
- Freshly ground black pepper, to taste

Directions:
- Combine the yogurt, parsley, lemon juice, garlic, salt, and a few grinds of black pepper in a medium-sized bowl.
- For up to five days, keep in the refrigerator in a sealed container.

NUTRITION FACTS:
- CALORIES: 24
- PROTEIN: 0g
- CARBS: 2g
- FAT: 2g

Remoulade

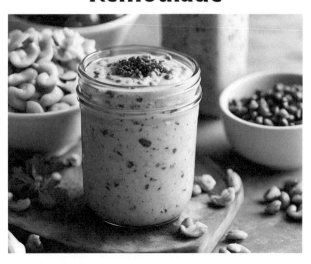

Makes: 1 cup

Ingredients:

- ½ cup raw cashews
- ½ cup plain, unsweetened almond milk
- 2 tablespoons ketchup
- 2 teaspoons brined capers
- 2 teaspoons caper brine
- 1 teaspoon Dijon mustard
- 1 teaspoon white vinegar
- ½ teaspoon sea salt
- ¼ teaspoon garlic powder
- 1 tablespoon sweet relish

Directions:

- Put the cashews, almond milk, vinegar, salt, garlic powder, ketchup, capers, and caper brine in a blender.
- Process till smooth. Fold in the relish with a spoon or spatula.
- For up to five days, keep in the refrigerator in a sealed container.

NUTRITION FACTS:

- CALORIES: 27
- PROTEIN: 1g
- CARBS: 2g
- FAT: 2g

Desdserts

Vanilla Tapioca Pudding

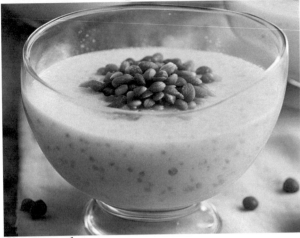

Serves: 1

Ingredients:

- 2 tablespoons tapioca pearls
- ¼ cup hot water
- 1 cup plain, unsweetened almond milk
- ½ teaspoon vanilla extract
- Pinch of ground cinnamon
- Stevia or monk fruit drops, to taste

Directions:

- Place the tapioca pearls in a small bowl and soak in the hot water for ten to fifteen minutes, or until the liquid is completely absorbed.
- Place the tapioca that has been soaked in water along with any leftover liquid in a small saucepan.
- Over medium-high heat, stir in the almond milk and bring to a boil.
- Bring the mixture to a strong simmer and stir continuously for three to five minutes, or until it thickens. Increase the heat a little bit if, after five minutes, the mixture hasn't thickened.
- Take the pot off of the heat and mix in the sweeteners, cinnamon, and vanilla extract, according to taste.
- Before serving, let the pudding to cool a little.

NUTRITION FACTS:

- CALORIES: 118
- PROTEIN: 1g
- CARBS: 22g
- FAT: 2g

One-Bowl Heavenly Banana Brownies

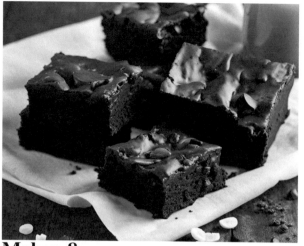

Makes: 8

Ingredients:

- Cooking spray
- 2 medium ripe bananas (194g)
- 2 tablespoons maple syrup
- 2 tablespoons unsweetened cocoa powder
- 1 teaspoon vanilla extract
- ½ cup gluten-free oat flour or regular all-purpose flour
- 1 teaspoon baking powder
- ⅛ teaspoon sea salt
- 2 tablespoons dairy-free chocolate chips

Directions:

- Set the oven's temperature to 375°F.
- Apply a thin layer of cooking spray to a loaf pan and place it aside.
- Mash the bananas with a fork in a medium-sized bowl until they are smooth and creamy.
- Combine the vanilla, cocoa powder, and maple syrup with the bananas and stir until everything is completely combined. Add the baking powder, salt, and oat flour, and stir until thoroughly mixed.
- Pour the batter into the pan that has been ready and level the top with a spatula.
- Over the batter, evenly distribute the chocolate chips.
- Bake for 18 to 20 minutes, or until the brownies are mostly set but still have some gooey middle when a knife is inserted.
- Avoid overbaking so as to prevent dry brownies.
- Cut into eight equal pieces and enjoy.
- Any leftover brownies can be frozen for up to two weeks or kept at room temperature for up to three days in an airtight container.

NUTRITION FACTS:

- CALORIES: 81
- PROTEIN: 2g
- CARBS: 13g
- FAT: 2g

Banana Crème Pie Pudding

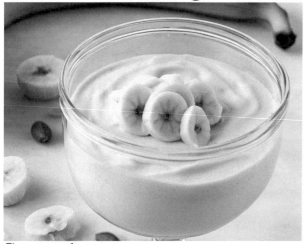

Serves: 1

Ingredients:

- 1 cup plain, unsweetened almond milk
- 1½ tablespoons corn-starch
- ¼ teaspoon banana extract
- ¼ teaspoon vanilla extract
- Stevia or monk fruit drops, to taste
- ½ medium banana (59g), sliced
- 3 tablespoons almond milk whipped cream

Directions:

- In a medium saucepan, mix the corn-starch and almond milk together, whisking until there are no lumps.
- Whisk continuously while heating the mixture over medium-high heat until it starts to boil.
- Lower the heat to a simmer and keep whisking for approximately one minute, or until the mixture thickens. Take the pan off of the heat.
- Add sweetener to taste and stir in the vanilla and banana extracts.
- Once the pudding is put together, serve it warm or let it cool for 20 minutes in the fridge. (It's best right after preparation.)
- Add the whipped cream and banana slices on top when you're ready to serve.

NUTRITION FACTS:

- CALORIES: 142
- PROTEIN: 2g
- CARBS: 28g
- FAT: 3g

Strawberry Shortcake

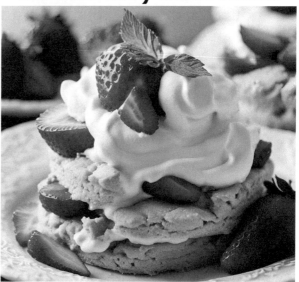

Serves: 2

Ingredients:

- 1 cup white whole-wheat flour
- 1 teaspoon baking powder
- ⅛ teaspoon sea salt
- ½ cup plus 2 tablespoons water
- ½ teaspoon vanilla extract
- 1 cup hulled and chopped fresh strawberries
- 3 tablespoons almond milk whipped cream

Directions:

- Set the oven's temperature to 375°F.
- Place parchment paper on a baking pan and set it aside.
- Using a small mixing bowl, thoroughly mix the flour, baking powder, and salt.
- Combine the vanilla and water in a measuring cup.
- While still whisking, slowly pour the vanilla mixture into the flour mixture.
- Use a spoon to stir the dough until it becomes homogenous after it starts to thicken.
- Form two biscuits of equal size using a ½-cup measuring cup.
- Spread out on the prepared baking sheet and bake for 10 to 12 minutes, or until they are

- just beginning to turn brown. Let them cool gently on the pan.
- Cut a slit along the center of each biscuit. Place a quarter of a cup of strawberries on the bottom side of each biscuit.
- Place the upper portion of the biscuit over the berries, then top with the whipped cream and the final ¼ cup of strawberries.

NUTRITION FACTS:

- CALORIES: 175
- PROTEIN: 6g
- CARBS: 30g
- FAT: 2g

Peaches and Cream

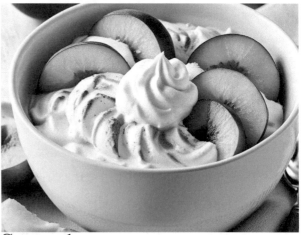

Serves: 1

Ingredients:

- 1 large ripe peach, pitted and cut into ½-inch-thick slices
- 1 teaspoon fresh lemon juice

- 1 teaspoon maple syrup
- 1 teaspoon vanilla extract
- Pinch of ground cinnamon
- Cooking spray
- 3 tablespoons almond milk whipped cream

Directions:
- Put the peach slices, lemon juice, maple syrup, cinnamon, and vanilla in a medium-sized bowl. Toss to coat.
- Add the peach mixture to a large, non-stick skillet that has been lightly sprayed with cooking spray.
- Simmer the peaches for approximately three minutes over medium heat, stirring once or twice, or until they start to get mushy and caramelized.
- Place the peaches in a serving bowl and top with the whipped cream before serving.

NUTRITION FACTS:
- CALORIES: 114
- PROTEIN: 2g
- CARBS: 20g
- FAT: 1g

Coffee-Chocolate Nice Cream

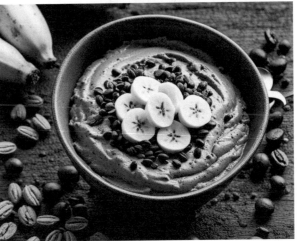

Serves: 1

Ingredients:
- 2 small bananas (200g), frozen and chopped
- ¼ cup plain, unsweetened almond milk
- ½ tablespoon instant coffee granules (I prefer decaf)
- 1 teaspoon vanilla extract
- 4 drops liquid stevia or monk fruit sweetener, plus more to taste
- ½ tablespoons dairy-free chocolate chips

Directions:
- Put the bananas, almond milk, instant coffee, vanilla, and sweetener in a food processor.
- Process the mixture until it resembles ice cream, stopping occasionally to use a spatula to

scrape down the sides of the bowl.

- Adjust sweetness as needed.
- Spoon the nice cream into a serving bowl, then sprinkle the chocolate pieces over it and serve.

NUTRITION FACTS:

- CALORIES: 251
- PROTEIN: 4g
- CARBS: 48g
- FAT: 4g

Coconut Banana Bites

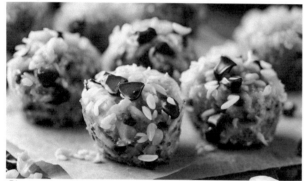

Serves: 5

Ingredients:

- 1 large banana (118g)
- 1 cup rolled oats
- 1 teaspoon vanilla extract
- 1 tablespoon shredded unsweetened coconut
- 2 tablespoons dairy-free chocolate chips

Directions:

- Set the oven's temperature to 375°F.
- Place parchment paper on a baking pan and set it aside.
- Mash the banana with a fork in a medium-sized bowl until it's almost smooth.
- Mix in the vanilla and oats, stirring until thoroughly combined.
- Divide the mixture into five tablespoon-sized portions, then place them in a single layer on the baking sheet that has been prepared.
- Shape each scoop into a doughnut-shaped cookie with your fingertips.
- Sprinkle grated coconut over the cookies and bake for approximately 10 minutes, or until the coconut has begin to brown.
- Leave the cookies on the pan to cool somewhat while you prepare the chocolate topping.
- Put the chocolate chips in a small bowl that can be microwaved.
- Heat for a total of one minute, stirring every twenty seconds, or until the chocolate is melted and smooth.
- Transfer the chocolate into a tiny plastic bag with a zip-top

and snip one corner.

- Drizzle each one with a little of chocolate.
- You can freeze leftover cookies for up to two weeks, or store them in an airtight jar at room temperature for up to five days.

NUTRITION FACTS:

- CALORIES: 123
- PROTEIN: 3g
- CARBS: 18g
- FAT: 4g

Cherry Pie Bowl

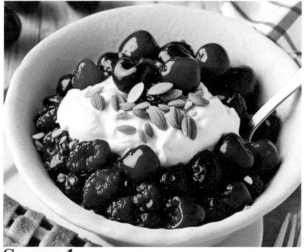

Serves: 1

Ingredients:

- 1 cup fresh cherries, pitted, or frozen cherries, thawed
- ¼ cup rolled oats
- ½ tablespoon maple syrup
- ¼ teaspoon vanilla extract
- ¼ teaspoon almond extract
- 2 tablespoons almond milk whipped cream

Directions:

- Set the oven's temperature to 400°F.
- Place the cherries in a small oven-safe dish and leave aside.
- Combine the oats, almond extract, vanilla, and maple syrup in a small bowl. Stir thoroughly to combine.
- Spoon the oat mixture over the cherries and bake for about 20 minutes, or until the oats start to brown and the cherries start to bubble.
- Let it cool down a little, then garnish with the whipped cream and serve warm.

NUTRITION FACTS:

- CALORIES: 210
- PROTEIN: 4g
- CARBS: 37g
- FAT: 2g

Acknowledgement

I would like to express my sincere gratitude to my friends, whose unwavering support and encouragement throughout this journey have been invaluable. Their belief in me and their willingness to taste-test my creations have been instrumental in bringing this cookbook to life.

I am also deeply indebted to the talented chefs who have inspired me with their culinary expertise and creativity. Their innovative recipes and techniques have enriched this cookbook and provided me with a wealth of knowledge.

A special thanks goes out to the dedicated editors who have meticulously shaped this book into its final form. Their keen eye for detail, their suggestions for improvement, and their commitment to excellence have been essential in ensuring the quality of this cookbook.

I am grateful to the talented photographers whose artistry has captured the essence of each dish. Their stunning images have brought the recipes to life, making this cookbook a visual delight.

Finally, I would like to thank all the readers who have supported me on this journey. Your enthusiasm and curiosity have motivated me to create this cookbook, and I hope that it will inspire you to embark on your own culinary adventures."

Made in the USA
Columbia, SC
05 October 2024

43636132R00043